ADVANCE PRAISE FOR

From Trauma to Healing

Dr. Lambert has been a subject-matter expert on trauma since the early 1990s. Her book is a wonderful, brilliant resource on the nature of trauma and the path to successful recovery. This book will be a treasured resource and companion for the individual trauma survivor, family members, physicians, trauma therapists, the clergy, and anyone wanting a deeper and nuanced understanding of the varied trauma experience, as well as paths towards recovery. Dr. Lambert guides us through the recovery process with clarity, very accessible content, and a wisdom evident in her courageous sharing of her own journey through trauma to a better place. The book reads as though you are having a safe, comfortable conversation with Dr. Lambert. In my 40 years of clinical practice and organizational consulting, this is the best book on trauma that I have ever read. You will come away with knowledge, a sense of purpose, and the seeds of a deep hope.

—Steven Flannes, PhD
Licensed Clinical Psychologist

As a primary care physician in practice for over 30 years, I often treat the symptoms of emotional trauma—heart palpitations, chest pain, depression, anxiety attacks, insomnia, nausea, diarrhea, and the like—rather than offering anything that's really effective at healing the wounds of trauma, other than time. Dr. Lambert's book spells out clear avenues to healing from deep trauma that are available to everyone, regardless of the type of trauma experienced or the sufferer's background or resources. Rather than relying on medications to relieve emotional and related physical pain and suffering, this book offers the reader roadmaps to transforming trauma to new and empowering perspectives, allowing us to regain control of fear, see obstacles as a means to new and valuable awareness, and imagine the possibilities of wholeness, acceptance, and unconditional love. Understanding how to redirect a life of fear, anger, and self-defeating thoughts into one of hope, balance, purpose, and peace may be just pages away.

—**James C. Gardner**, MD, Author
Overcoming Anxiety, Panic and Depression:
New Ways to Regain Your Confidence (2000),
Phobias and How to Overcome Them:
Understanding and Beating Your Fears (2005),
and *The Anxiety Toolbox Program:*
The Comprehensive, Integrative Approach
to Overcoming Anxious Emotions (2017)

In the somewhat crowded field of trauma literature, Dr. Lambert's book stands out for being personal, accessible, and educational. She carries us through the essence of various therapeutic modalities through the story of her own healing journey, and shares this with a vulnerability and transparency that is both compelling and inspirational.

—**Philip Brooks**, Ed.D.
Associate Professor, School of Professional Psychology and Health
California Institute of Integral Studies/ICP

Outstanding. Bobbi Lambert draws upon personal experience and 35 years as a consultant to provide helpful advice on grief and healing after unimaginable tragedy. Thoughtful, sensitive, moving, spiritual, practical, and, above all, hopeful. Highly recommended.

—**Sheldon Siegel**, Survivor of the 101 California Street shooting and *New York Times* bestselling author of the *Mike Daley/Rosie Fernandez* series of novels

It has truly been my honor and pleasure to accompany Dr. Bobbi Lambert over the course of several years following the passing of her mother. From the very beginning of our work together, I was struck by Bobbi's courage to explore challenging and painful inner territory. Bobbi's education and her abundant professional and personal life experience shine in this book. She examines deeply human experiences with her uniquely inspiring way of connecting the dots across the disciplines of psychology, psychosynthesis, trauma work, and systemic family dynamics (to name but a few). I trust you will come away as profoundly enriched from reading this enlightening and intimate examination of the human condition as I have been by witnessing one exceptional and graceful woman walk her talk with vulnerability and integrity.

—**Gita V. Wagner**, LMT, Somatic and Systemic Coach, certified life coach, and mindfulness retreat leader at MiiAmo Spa, Sedona, Arizona

Dr. Lambert offers a map of transformational healing for anyone who has endured trauma and wonders if there is a way to a fuller and healthier life on the other side. Walking the reader through the horrific big and little traumas of her own life gives the reader a deeper understanding of the many faces of present and ancestral trauma that can define and paralyze our lives. Determined to heal, Dr. Lambert courageously takes the longest journey from head to heart as she unpacks her own trauma and offers us a step-by-step guide that invites the reader to a fuller life of improved health, unconditional love, deeper connections, and a legacy of hope for the future. Without reservation, I recommend this book to my patients and parishioners!

—**Danielle Green**, PhD, Psychoanalyst, Marriage and Family Therapist, Ordained Unitarian Universalist Minister

In *From Trauma to Healing*, Dr. Lambert bravely takes a deep dive into her own Big Trauma and extensive academic and nationally recognized professional career to provide the reader a pathway for discovery and ultimately recovery of a safe and fulfilling life. Lambert thoughtfully offers sage advice on retrieving lost elements of hope and even prospering from life's tragedies towards meaningful change, growth, and trust. She underscores a key to healing: finding a safe, emotional connection in another to help dissolve both learned and self-destructive fear. An essential read not only for clinicians and threat assessment and human resource professionals, but for those seeking escape from the cycle of despair.

—**Robert L. Weisman**, DO, Professor of Psychiatry, Director, Fellowship in Psychiatry and Law, University of Rochester Medical Center

from trauma to
healing

SEEKING SOLACE AND
SAFE PLACES TO FALL

DR. BOBBI LAMBERT

modern wisdom
PRESS

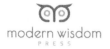

Modern Wisdom Press Boulder,
Colorado, USA
www.modernwisdompress.com

Published 2020
Cover Design: Karen Sperry Design
Author's photo courtesy of Susan Adler

DISCLAIMER

Neither the author nor the publisher assumes any responsibility for errors, omissions, or contrary interpretations of the subject matter within.

This book includes the truthful recollection of actual events in my life. The following account reflects my own personal remembrances of the private and public experiences that have shaped my life. Some names and characteristics have been changed, some events have been compressed, and some dialogue has been recreated. Others may have different memories of events, and they are welcome to write their own accounts. The case studies in the book are based on actual events. In order to protect the identities of those concerned, names and personal details have been altered where necessary.

MEDICAL DISCLAIMER

The information in this book is a result of years of practical experience by the author. This information is not intended as a substitute for the advice provided by your physician or other healthcare professional. Do not use the information in this book for diagnosing or treating a health problem or disease, or prescribing medication or other treatment.

Dedication

For Norm, whose unconditional love and love of writing taught me how to express what is in my heart and find the sanctuary I've always sought.

And to my children, Debbie and Marc, and my grandchildren, Kelsey, Matt, Mason, Lauryn, and Francesca: May your lives be filled with unconditional love and safe places to fall. Thank you all for blessing my life, each in your own unique way.

And finally to my dad, Eddie, who lost his life so long ago, yet continues to inspire me to live my best life and always reach for the stars.

Contents

Foreword

I AM HONORED TO WRITE THIS FOREWORD FOR DR. BOBBI LAMBERT. I am in a unique position to tell you about the author of this excellent book, her quest for healing trauma, and the many forms it takes and its effects on the human psyche.

Bobbi and I first met over 40 years ago and received much of our formal training together. We became classmates shortly after she suffered a major life trauma that propelled her to not only seek her own healing but to learn to help others. I was inspired as I watched her journey to recovery. This book is her gift to all of us who have suffered or are suffering the aftereffects of trauma, as Dr. Lambert artfully lays out universal trauma truths and guides us on the path to healing.

Dr. Lambert and I became friends and colleagues over the years. We offered each other personal and professional support and guidance. We visited the red rock canyons outside Sedona together and provided each other with solace and safe places to become more and more authentic in our personal and professional lives. I have personal insight into the quality of her professional work with clients and of Bobbi as a person. She is the calm we want with us in the storms we weather in life.

From Trauma to Healing: Seeking Solace and Safe Places to Fall is a powerful reading experience that is filled with provocative stories and intriguing theoretical approaches to healing trauma rarely explained in such a practical and accessible way. Dr. Lambert's compassionate and tender voice, which I have experienced conversationally over the years, flows through her words as she shares her extraordinary life experiences and directly addresses you, her reader. You will find healing in her wisdom. Her insights and advice will provide you with new knowledge regarding the known and unknown consequences of trauma that may be actively at play in your day-to-day life, but that do not have to continue to be.

In my professional research and work, I have conducted many interviews with children of different cultures throughout the world, all of whom demonstrate the universal trait of innate wisdom. Throughout this book, Dr. Lambert speaks eloquently to the wisdom of the child within each of us and to the adults we are constantly becoming.

Perhaps, most importantly, she will become your advocate and provide a safe place for you as she guides you deeper into yourself than you imagine a book has the power to do. She is a trustworthy friend and a respected professional in her chosen career, working with partnerships, large and small corporations, and non-profit organizations that touch others. Bobbi Lambert offers a unique perspective and experience base that you won't find elsewhere. She has a deep understanding of human behavior and by bravely using her own journey of healing as an example throughout these pages, she leads us to better understand why we do the things we do even as we continue to re-injure ourselves.

I have also watched Bobbi's willingness to be transformed in the process of writing this book. If my writing career inspired hers, I am grateful that she persevered and know that you will be the beneficiary of her authentic and insightful writing.

Her light shines into the shadowy corners of our psyches, making it safer for us to explore and to shed the remnants of trauma that have lived in the darkness too long undermining our sense of wellbeing and self-love. With this beautiful book, Dr. Lambert provides you, the reader, with welcoming sanctuary in uncertain times and teaches you of the power of unconditional love.

—**Dr. Emma Farr Rawlings**
Author of *The Divine Child: Your Soul's Inner Voice*
Psychotherapist, ICF Master Certified Coach, Humanitarian and Advocate for Children (www.thedivinechild.org)

Introduction

I AUTHORED THIS BOOK BECAUSE I HAVE SO MUCH TO SHARE WITH you. As an expert in human behavior, I have had a long, busy, and unique career assisting people to confront trauma, many of whom were hanging by a burning thread on the edge of life-changing events. I will give you just two examples.

In 1993, I was the lead crisis counselor during one of the nation's first mass workplace shootings, which took place at the law offices of Pettit & Martin at 101 California Street in the heart of San Francisco's financial district. I could hear the shots being fired and the panic that resulted while I was on the phone with the human resources manager. In the aftermath, I was there to support the survivors, some who were wounded, to regain their feelings of safety and normality.

In the 1980s, I cared for and counseled teams of caregivers suffering through feelings of helplessness and sorrow as their young and healthy patients were attacked and killed by the HIV/AIDS epidemic. I also helped loved ones say goodbye.

In part, I believe I was especially qualified to care for and calm others because I too knew exactly how they were feeling. I gained this insight the hard way when the father I dearly loved was murdered in our San Francisco neighborhood in 1976.

In the aftermath of my own personal "burning thread," I pledged to myself that I would learn everything I possibly could about human behavior—from the ruthless worst among us to helping others find and achieve the beauty and comfort of unconditional love.

I earned two post-graduate degrees in psychology, studying the works of the world's finest behavioral scholars. In 1982, I launched a lifelong career as a counselor and consultant, helping people heal from traumatic and life-altering events.

We have all experienced traumatic events. If you were lucky, yours were small. If they were big ones, they probably sent you on an urgent search for a safe place. I have included in this book examples of how you might find sanctuaries—real and metaphorical—where you can fall and recover and the tools to help you do so.

What follows is my unfolding story in search of truth, along with struggles, setbacks, insights, and theories that explain the mysteries of human behavior to help you on your own journey. I'll also explore the ways in which the past influences the present. I hope my story as well as the reader activities and questioning throughout will be an inspiration to you.

PART I

What Is Trauma?

CHAPTER 1

Trauma and You

"Who looks outside, dreams; who looks inside, awakens."

—CARL GUSTAV JUNG

TRAUMA TRANSFORMS US. I KNOW BECAUSE I WAS TRANSFORMED BY the murder of my father. That event ignited my determined quest to understand the aftereffects of trauma that turned my life upside down. Preventing others from suffering the unseen effects of trauma has been a professional commitment and a personal one. But I'll tell you my story later.

What does the term "trauma" mean to you? And what does it have to do with who you are today or why you are reading this book now? I don't know your story, but you may be concerned that shocking and painful—perhaps devastating—events that you have endured are impacting your peace of mind, sense of safety, health, or relationships in negative ways. Perhaps you realize that your traumas are affecting you in ways that you don't even fully understand.

The consequences of trauma never really disappear. They slide below the surface of our awareness and we go on with our lives, yet their impact is often life-changing and mind-numbing. Making the crucial connections between painful past experiences and current problems can help you now and lead to positive changes in your future.

Do you avoid intimacy? Or do you choose the same damaging types of relationships over and over again? Are your buried emotions contributing to or causing physical illness? Do you have one abusive boss after another? Do you engage in self-sabotaging behaviors that you can't seem to change despite your best efforts? Were you the victim of some form of abuse, and do you recognize any abusive behaviors in yourself?

Wherever you are in your life, whatever problems you have faced, whatever challenges you may be facing now, there's hope. Sharing the hard lessons we learn from surviving traumatic events can be cathartic and healing. I imagine, whatever your story, you have something to teach me about trauma and survival. And I believe there are things I can teach you. If I can help you through the pages of this book by sharing the wisdom I've gained through lived experience and while counseling others, then all the trials and tribulations, ups and downs, losses and gains will take on new meaning.

Trauma Defined

Allow me to explain to you my understanding, personally and professionally, of trauma and its wide-ranging impact, causes, and effects. Ultimately, trauma—like beauty—is in the eye of the beholder. Like grief, it is suffered in ways that are unique to each of us, although the stages we go through have similarities. Each of us has a singular path to healing. Yet, again, the components of healing are universal and, I believe, attainable.

Would it surprise you, for instance, to know that 70 percent of adults in the United States have experienced some type of traumatic event at least once in their lives, according to the National Council for Behavioral Health? In its 2015 study, 61 percent of men and 57 percent of women reported exposure to at least one traumatic event in their lifetimes. Those statistics are startling, but I don't believe they fully represent the unseen, widespread, and long-lasting nature of the psychological and emotional injuries most of us have suffered repeatedly in our lives.

Trauma is often defined as a deeply disturbing and distressing experience or injury and the emotional shock that accompanies it. The Big Traumas we often think of are those that involve natural disasters, accidents, wars, violence, and sexual or non-sexual assaults that result in serious physical injuries or death.

There are other traumas that don't necessarily result in physical damage. They involve repetitive, ongoing psychological and emotional injuries that we suffer at the hands of family members, intimate partners, or bullies at work or school. And there are inherited traumas that pass from one generation to the next.

For the most part, generational trauma occurs unconsciously. Many people are not aware that their present-day traumas have often been passed down from their ancestors. Yet this suffering that replays over time can have the power to impact the roles we play and the bonds we share with family members in present day.

At the time of writing this book, in the year 2020, I would add the traumatic outbreak of the COVID-19 pandemic to the list of traumas outlined above. The scale of this event is beyond comprehension at this time. It is causing Big Trauma around the world in the form of livelihoods lost, illness, hospitalization, and death.

Current events also have the power to reawaken past fears and trauma that we may have thought we had put to rest. They also test coping mechanisms that we believed served us but no longer do.

Would you place yourself or anyone close to you among the unfortunate 70th percentile of major traumatic event sufferers? Have you experienced some level of trauma, big or small, in a single event or over an extended period? Would you include yourself among the countless millions of people around the world who have felt the traumatic impact of the 2020 pandemic? If so, then this book is for you.

It is important to note that trauma, in all its forms, is often the root cause of many emotional, psychological, health, and relationship problems that impact us in unknown and unseen ways. Trauma also causes people to turn to alcohol or drug abuse to escape or numb themselves to their suffering.

One of the important goals of this book is to assure you that the impact of your trauma can be effectively balanced. In my case, it actually motivated me to do the work that resulted in my professional career in helping others heal from their traumatic events. I hope by sharing what I've learned over my 35-year career as a human behavior expert, executive coach, and consultant, I can support you on your path to healing from your own history of trauma.

Recognizing and reconciling the lingering effects of trauma on your health, happiness, relationships, safety, and well-being is the first important step toward positive change. Understanding the emotional impact of past traumas that create day-to-day feelings of anxiety, anger, depression, or hopelessness will help you begin to regain control of your life.

I'd love for you to be able to say, "I'm no longer held back by the painful events in my past, and I am thriving and in control of my own destiny." With this book, you've taken the first step toward making that dream come true.

Safe Places to Fall

Trauma's grip on us can be paralyzing, freezing every part of our being into inaction. Most of us feel unsafe at one time or another. Yet feeling safe within ourselves and with the people we relate to is one of our most basic biological and human emotional needs. Most of us have lost love, whether through broken relationships, death, or alienation from family members. Broken hearts, hardships, and drama, large or small, can throw an orderly life into chaos.

Loosening the hold of trauma and gaining confidence to relax into the arms of unconditional love for self and others is the freedom essential to our healing. Having safe places to fall and people who provide sanctuary for you in good times and bad is crucial. It is one of the most powerful antidotes, along with unconditional love, to apply to the traumas we have experienced.

A safe place to fall, in my experience, is both an internal and external "place." It is a location where we feel safe, comfortable, calm, accepted, and supported. It may be a physical environment, whether among the red rocks of the high desert, at the beach, or in the mountains beside a deep, clear lake fed by melting snow, where you feel the peace and calm in yourself and your surroundings. It can be an environment where you think clearly, gain perspective, renew faith, and take a deep breath. There is the feeling of being at home and of home being your sanctuary. It's safe in this place, whether you're alone there or in the company of your safe people. This is something you have the capacity to access for yourself.

Safe places to fall alone are illuminated by the unconditional love we can learn to feel for ourselves. Finding solace and peace inside may be the greatest gift you could give to yourself and others in your life. This is where we find balance and strength, where we can tell ourselves the truth and be unafraid of what we hear. In these interior safe places, we can give expression to our deepest desires, enjoy our own company, and even learn to laugh at ourselves.

With others, our safe places to fall are the relationships—whether with friends, intimate partners, or family members—where love flows without condition. These are involvements with the people who understand, accept, and respect us. We can tell our truths, share our emotions, and find solace and support. We feel heard.

Actions, words, facial expressions, and body language consistently tell us we are safe. In safe relationships, we can lower our defenses and allow ourselves to be more vulnerable. These connections with others are marked by consistency: *I know you have my back. I know what to expect. You help me believe in the inherent goodness in myself and others. The look in your eyes tells me you love me. The sound of your voice is patient and kind even when you tell me something I may not want to hear but need to.*

Imagine falling into the outstretched arms of 100,000 angels, as one of my favorite songs by a group called Bliss suggests. Imagine collapsing into the arms of an unconditionally loving and trusted partner. Or imagine closing the door and entering the sanctuary of home after a harrowing day, settling into the silence and comfort you have with yourself.

My definition of safe places differs greatly from designated "safe spaces" like the ones that have been established at colleges and universities. Those are temporary escapes from the challenges of life. You don't take that feeling of safety with you when you leave because you generally don't internalize it.

If you want to truly heal from trauma, creating genuine safe places to fall will allow you to do just that.

Self-Reflection and Healing

Would you say, right now, that you are at peace with yourself? Are your relationships harmonious? Are you at peace with the role you play in your family and the role family members play in your life? Are you healthy or do you face health challenges that may be rooted in past trauma? Have you recovered from a serious illness but fear there will be a next time? And are you in an unconditionally loving and nonjudgmental relationship, or do you long for one?

I am filled with questions like these for you that are not unlike those I have asked myself, clients, and friends over and over again. If I had not opened up my mind and faced some of my worst fears and deepest truths, I would not have the peace of mind and unconditional love I have today.

I hope you read these words with an open mind, an open heart, and the belief that life is a continuous learning ground filled with opportunity. I hope you believe you can free yourself from past and present trauma. I hope you realize the dreams you have put aside and learned to live without.

I want to help you find your happy ending, but let's be clear. There is no easy way out here. The healing process will take effort on your part. You will stay in relationships or jobs that you should leave until you find the strength within to do so. You will stumble and fall as we all do. There are no shortcuts to healing. You will get frustrated along the way, but don't give up. Living in the shadow of trauma is not a life sentence. You can break free of the past. Embarking on the journey may be one of the greatest gifts you can give to yourself.

In the chapters that follow, I share my story and the stories of people I have had the honor to work with and learn from. I also include psychological theories and research that you can apply to your own life that will help explain the influence of trauma and illuminate the path to healing.

Together, we can unravel some of the confusing complexities that drive human behavior. This knowledge and suggestions for their practical application in your life can help you navigate the unconscious drivers, repressed emotions, and unseen forces that influence your life in unhealthy and self-defeating ways. As you learn to face your past traumas and buried emotions and confront the unhealthy patterns, circumstances, and people in your life, you will be able to live life more fully, freely, and lovingly.

Throughout the coming pages, you'll find questions and suggestions that I hope will serve as a roadmap to your self-inquiry and breakthrough discoveries. After all, how many of us can honestly say there is no more healing to be done? I know I can't. No matter how far I have come, I am always humbled to discover there is more healing to be done on my journey through life. I choose to keep going. Whatever you choose to take from this journey we are embarking on in this book is up to you; however you choose to apply what you uncover is in your hands.

CHAPTER 2

My Journey

*"The reality is that you will grieve forever. You will not 'get over' the loss
of a loved one; you will learn to live with it. You will heal and
you will rebuild yourself around the loss you have suffered.
You will be whole again but you will never be the same."*

—ELIZABETH KUBLER-ROSS

FOR MANY OF US, IT IS TRAUMA THAT FORCES US ONTO THE PATH OF
healing. Trauma can break us in ways that make recovery seem
impossible. That's how it feels. The world is shattered, and we are
left to face an unrecognizable reality. Nothing will be the same
again. We won't be the same.

While I could tell you that my education and graduate degrees in
psychology qualify me to guide you on your journey from trauma to
healing, it is important that you know that my personal experience
and recovery propelled me to heal others.

So that you understand who I am and what I bring to the subject
matter at the heart of this book, I will share with you my major life
trauma, or what I call the Big Trauma. To give context and perspective to this central event, I will also offer a brief history of the family
dysfunction and trauma that robbed me of a safe place to fall at
times in my life when I needed it most.

The Big Trauma

I don't know how my life would have unfolded if my world had not been smashed into millions of tiny shards by a fusillade of gunfire that I didn't even hear. There are events that happen in your life that you will always remember and forever wish you could forget. There are events that take place that destroy your life as you know it and render what was unrecoverable.

The belief system you utilized to understand the world you live in is turned inside out and upside down. Faith is demolished. Religious beliefs fail you. Support systems constructed to sustain you let you down. Sanctuary no longer exists; there is no escape. Suddenly you are filled with terrifying thoughts and truths you can't escape. My Big Trauma started with a late-night phone call, one of those calls you never want to receive.

Let me introduce you to Eddie, my father. He was a handsome man, six feet four tall. He was healthy, fit, and successful. He was confident. He was also complex, as was our relationship with one another. He wore a watch fob on a chain clipped to a belt loop on the waist of his custom-tailored suit pants; his diamond Star of David hung there too.

Dad was a proud Jew, a huge supporter of the State of Israel. He was the son of Russian immigrants who fled their native country to avoid religious persecution and almost certain death. He suffered cruel acts of anti-Semitism growing up outside Portland, Oregon, and never forgot.

We worked together in his insurance business in San Francisco. Our offices at 50 Francisco Street were graced with a magnificent water view of the San Francisco Bay Area. On Friday, November 19, 1976, Dad left the office at noon as he often did.

It was the day before the annual big game between Stanford and his alma mater, Cal Berkeley. I was the third generation of Cal attendees. My parents met there in the early 1930s and my great uncle, Rube Goldberg, the famous Pulitzer Prize-winning cartoonist, graduated from there at the turn of the 20th century.

As always, that day Dad was upbeat when he was bound for 18 holes of golf, especially on big game weekend. I kissed him on the cheek on his way out. We shared a long hug and promised to see each other for a family dinner that was scheduled for Sunday night.

Dad was still young to me in his mid-60s. His new pacemaker made him more energetic. He now had a good chance for a long and healthy life. I looked forward to sharing it with him. And then, the next day, everything changed forever, without any warning at all.

It was 10 p.m. on Saturday, November 20, 1976, after Cal lost a close game to Stanford. According to a time-honored tradition, my parents attended the game, followed by a party given by my cousins.

Upon returning home, my parents, as was their habit, clipped a leash to the collar of our black miniature poodle, Pepper. Dad closed the automatic garage door and they headed up Clay Street to the corner of Maple, the beginning of their usual route.

I do not doubt that Dad walked proudly, straight and tall, and unafraid, casting an impressive shadow on the sidewalk from the many streetlights that illuminated their stroll. As my parents crossed Maple and turned to walk toward Washington, they couldn't know they would be rapidly intercepted by four dark and hooded figures.

One of these young men, like the alpha in a pride of lions, darted out of the dark, the others following close behind. As my mother later described it, my parents were suddenly surrounded. Out of the pitch blackness that hooded his head came the hard voice of the leader, "Give up your money, you fucking old man."

In the night, my parents couldn't see the weapon in his hand. My mother immediately retrieved her small evening bag from her coat pocket and found the few dollars within it, throwing them down on the sidewalk at his feet. One of the others snatched them up.

My father moved forward to protect my mother, but his motion was halted. He was thrown to the ground by the force of two bullets fired at close range. One hit him in the head, the other in his liver, but according to my mother, he was still conscious and breathing.

Mom screamed and ran for help as the exhilarated pack sprinted away in the direction from which they had come, laughing. Pepper bolted for home, dragging his leash behind him. At that point, my mother ran up the stairs of the big brick house on the corner, near the mailbox where Dad lay bleeding. Although the lights in the house were on and the doctor and his family who lived there were home, they didn't respond to her repeated knocking or cries for help.

In fact, Mom later told me that she was so frantic that she kicked at their door with the heel of her shoe with all the force she could gather. She finally gave up and ran to the house across the street where she found help and access to a phone. She called the police and had an ambulance dispatched and then called me.

When I put the receiver to my ear, it was my mother's voice quivering like I never heard it before. And then, without warning, she unleashed a torrent of words that stunned me to the point that I suddenly needed to swivel the kitchen chair around and sit down.

Mom said, "Dad's been shot. He's lying on the sidewalk." She was hysterical. I was struggling to understand her, let alone absorb what she was saying. I tried to calm her down but couldn't. She said, "The gun was so loud, we didn't even see it except when it was fired, and the noise was so loud. There was so much blood."

Through her tears, I could hear her say, "They took Dad away but they wouldn't let me go with him. Dad was calling my name, begging me not to leave him alone. They told me it was a police matter and they were taking him to San Francisco General Hospital." Then she cried and said, "Honey, come get me right away. We need to go to your father."

To this day, the memories of that night remain crystal clear. They roll through my mind like the familiar scenes of a movie on an endless loop that I can't stop. I see myself standing up, rising from the kitchen chair where I sat to stabilize myself during Mom's call.

When I turned around, I saw my husband Jason and my children from my first marriage standing in the kitchen, eyes locked on me, their arms around each other. And then, somehow, we kicked into high gear even though everything else seemed to be moving in slow motion.

The four of us piled into our station wagon. In less than five minutes, we were gathering Mom into the car from the spot where she stood waiting on the sidewalk with the neighbors who had been kind enough to take her in.

Clay Street was ablaze with flashing lights. Crime scene chalk outlined where my father's body had fallen. Armed detectives were combing the neighborhood for clues. Onlookers were gathering. We, however, had no time to waste. We raced across town, passing two private hospitals within blocks of our family home that could have meant the difference between life and death. Somehow, in a matter of minutes, my father became the victim of a crime—a police matter that seemed to be a higher priority than fighting for his life.

My mother's words still haunt me. "They slammed the ambulance doors in my face. He's alone. It's so bad." And then: "Why didn't they shoot me too?"

And the possibility that this night could somehow be worse sank us into a deeper silence, only broken by the opening and closing of the car doors as we exited the car. We entered the emergency waiting room at San Francisco General Hospital, which might as well have been the far side of the moon—if not, then the depths of hell. My psyche, at that moment, was under attack by wave after wave of Big Trauma.

We were crammed into a glass-enclosed room that filled rapidly with family members as word spread like wildfire. Police and doctors came and went. All we were told was that Dad was alive and in surgery.

An hour later, the immediate family was taken up in a service elevator to the surgery floor. We were ushered into a larger, more comfortable waiting room. All I wanted was to see Dad, to hold his hand, to kiss his forehead. I wanted to let him know that we were there. Instead, we waited, and the police began to interrogate my mother. The scene was surreal. She was the only eyewitness, and they wanted any information she could provide them while the scene was fresh in her mind.

Then the surgeons came into the room in their scrubs to tell us of another delay. Because of the pacemaker that had been implanted in Dad's heart, the trauma surgeons now needed to locate and wait for a heart surgeon to arrive before they could remove the bullet lodged in his liver. Ironically, my Dad's heart surgeon lived on Clay Street, less than two blocks from where he had been shot.

I couldn't help but think that if Mom were in that ambulance with Dad she would have told the EMTs that his surgeon was on the staff of Mt. Zion Hospital, just five minutes away. Instead, police protocol, not medical protocol, mandated a 45-minute ambulance ride rather than a quick delivery to Mt. Zion that might have saved Dad's life.

Now we were being told by the surgeons that we should trek completely across the city again and just wait at home for their call. They said it could be a long night and that we would not be able to see him even if we stayed. I was reluctant to leave, but they left us with no choice.

We returned to 7th Avenue in the middle of the night. The house filled with family and religious leaders; two rabbis came to pray for Dad. Within the hour the phone rang. This time when I picked it up, what I feared came: "I'm sorry to tell you your father died on the operating table a short time ago. We did our best, but we lost him." I laid the phone down on the counter and repeated the news to my family. Then the blinding tears began to fall.

Sometimes now at night I hear the yipping and howling of a pack of coyotes as they gather for their nightly hunt in the oak woods that surround my house. Every time I listen to their shrill and haunting calls, I am reminded of the harsh demands of the pack of animals that gathered in the shadows and emerged to rip my world apart and rob me of my father's love. I had no idea whether I could survive a world without my father in it or if I would even want to.

That call and its aftermath very nearly destroyed me. I still shake with fear if the phone rings late at night. If someone I love or work with calls me and I hear the sound of panic in their voice, I dread the worst. But that night, I had no idea that just about everything in my life would be changed forevermore. I also didn't know that the trauma and drama of my early years would haunt and injure me in new ways that deepened my psychological and emotional pain over many decades.

Repetitive Trauma

Dad's passing brought to light the ongoing trauma that I experienced in my family but had never really dealt with. I could not measure the impact of it fully until Dad was no longer there to protect me and create a zone of safety within which I could grow.

Many of you may have suffered trauma that was repetitive, either because of family dynamics; a troubling, abusive personal relationship; or a workplace situation in which you were subjected to bullying or harassment regularly. Perhaps you didn't understand at the time just how unhealthy the situation was for you, or maybe escape wasn't viable, as in the case of a child.

During a major trauma, when we need others most and we turn to the people who surround us at home or work, we sometimes discover the support we need is not there. The negative effects of trauma are compounded and made worse because of the lack of a healthy support system and the absence of unconditional love. There may be no safe place for our suffering.

When Dad died, I felt alone in my grief, though I was surrounded by family. It was only then that I came to accept how much I had been impacted over my life by the dysfunction I was born into. Dad's loss laid bare the failings of our family unit and his role in it. One painful event unmasked another.

I grew up with the advantages others dream of. I had the physical comforts I needed. I was never physically abused. I suffered no real tragedies or losses. I had much to be grateful for. It was only later that I gained insight into family tensions and came to fully understand the negative effect that the absence of unconditional love and close family bonds can have on a child.

It seemed instead, in my experience, that love was given or taken away on a whim, creating an environment of instability. I never really felt at home or learned to become part of a family that was rooted in discord, competition, and jealousy. It was my father's love, imperfect as it was, and my dependence on the family unit that kept me there until he no longer was.

When I was born, I immediately became new competition for the love and attention that my brother, sister, and mother craved from Dad. They wanted his time, they wanted his affection, and they had neither. He gave me what they wanted from him. Looking back, I think Dad took pleasure using me to irritate the other family members. Whenever he could, he would take me on special adventures, leaving the others behind.

My mother, Dottie, and sister, Ann, came to view me as "the other woman" in Dad's life and weren't shy about implying that. My brother, Garry, the middle child, was already suffering from the discord when I was born. Mostly, he tried to stay out of everyone's way.

When I was in my teens, my sister's disturbing view of my relationship with Dad spilled out while my first boyfriend was having dinner at our house. Out of the blue, Ann blurted out, "They have an incestuous relationship, you know. I'd be very careful if I were you."

My parents' reaction stunned me almost as much as Ann's remark. My mother sat at the end of the white marble dining room table with a polite smile on her face. Even Dad didn't admonish my sister; he tried to laugh it off as if she were just joking. She wasn't.

Even though I suffered the consequences of being Dad's favorite, I adored the time, love, and attention he gave me. The scorn and contempt of my mother and sister seemed worth it somehow. I couldn't give up the only safe place I had within the family unit.

When I joined the family as the third and youngest child, I was given the smallest room in the farthest corner in a large and imposing three-story house. I was often left to cry in my crib. The saving grace was when the door to my room would open softly in the early hours of the morning and Dad would pick me up, hold me close, and whisper, "Good morning, baby." In those moments, I felt safe and calm until he put me back into my crib, quietly closed the door behind him, and left for work before anyone else in the house stirred.

Mom and Dad lacked compatibilities and "other women" were how my father made up for what was missing in their union. He loved the respectability that came from their marriage and position in the community. Divorce wasn't an option. But sides were clearly drawn in our family. I was on Dad's side. My sister and brother were on Mom's side.

As I grew up, when we were all in the house, what I remember most is the anger and resentment that often swirled around me. I hated the screaming and yelling and wild accusations that were thrown about. My mother and sister were angry screamers. I went the other way and rarely allowed myself to feel any anger at all. Instead, I felt the pain of the hostility around me.

I would run and hide in my bed to escape the loud and emotional clashes, often centered on Dad's most recent girlfriend. In those moments, I was grateful for the smallest room in the farthest corner of the large house.

My mother was distant, dismissive, and cold. She always seemed to be mad at me for something. She'd yell at Dad, "She's your daughter. You wanted her. I didn't. You take care of it. I'm done with her."

My friends and I were afraid of my sister, especially if we were left in her care. As I grew older, I realized that love didn't flow naturally in our family as I imagined it must in other families.

The Trauma of Rejection

A critical turning point in my early life was the rejection of me by Dad. As I said, my father had a complex personality, and in some ways, he was deeply flawed. Still, I needed to see him as my protector and guardian.

In 1963, while studying at the University of Arizona, where I had transferred from Berkeley, I discovered that I was pregnant. I was terrified but committed to having my baby and marrying her father, Glen, who I had known for three months.

When I came home for Christmas break, I told Dad of my predicament that morning. "Well," Dad said, "I'll send you to another doctor who I know and he'll help us. You'll get an abortion while you're home and go right back to school after New Year's."

When I told him my baby's life was more important than any future plans we had made or our family's reputation, his face was a mixture of disbelief and anger. He asked, "How do you plan to deal with this dilemma since you will be dealing with it on your own? It appears there is nothing I can say that will change your mind."

And then, without a hint of love or compassion, he said, "You are not welcome in this house or family until and unless you come to your senses. You can take your car and whatever cash is in your savings account. Leave your Star of David and your credit cards. I expect you to be gone before I get home tonight."

I learned at that moment that Dad's love for me was not unconditional. If it had been, he would have embraced and comforted, not rejected, me and my baby. At that moment, I understood how it feels to have a broken heart. I did leave home later that day. Glen and I got married in Reno and moved to the Bay Area, where we got jobs. The only family support we received was from my maternal grandmother, Hazel. She was unrelenting in her efforts to "talk sense" into my parents.

Finally, they gave in and Glen and I moved back into my old bedroom in the house on Clay Street. A month later, we welcomed a beautiful baby into the world. My estrangement from my family didn't last long and was rarely mentioned again. I buried the pain of rejection and desperately tried to act like the disowning never happened. My daughter was welcomed into the family and became a well-cared-for and loved insider, while I tried to fit in but never succeeded.

I did later recover my relationship with Dad and earn his respect and admiration once again. I accepted the love he had to give. I didn't judge it and I certainly did not want to risk losing it again. I was also blessed by the birth of my second child, a son, born four years later. My marriage to Glen, however, ended in divorce six years after it began, breaking under the pressure of our premature union and mounting responsibilities.

This time, Dad was there to help me get back on my feet and to love my children. I got on with my life, went to work for Dad, and gave up dreams of going back to school. Several years later, my second husband, Jason, and I were married. We settled into a comfortable rhythm that lasted until the night Dad died.

Life after Loss

After losing my father, I did go back to school to finish my bachelor's degree and earn two graduate degrees in psychology. I dedicated myself to researching and learning everything I could about grief, loss, and trauma and its impact on human behavior. I went on to become a nationally recognized expert on workplace violence.

I have spent over 35 years working in this field, at first independently, then within two major companies in the health care arena, before cofounding my own consulting company, Confidante, Inc., with my partner, Norm. Our business is still flourishing today.

I am motivated by the traumas that deeply impacted me and those of others whom I worked with over the years. I am inspired by the opportunity to prevent others from suffering similarly when proactive measures are possible. When there is danger, I seek to find safety. When there is discord, I seek harmony. When there is trauma, I set about the process of recovery and healing.

I don't believe that I am alone on my path to healing and helping others. While trauma has the power to shake us to the core and render the thought of recovery a near-impossible task, somehow we find our way. So often, and gratefully, we are able to take the painful experiences that happen to us and use them to provide sanctuary and safety to others similarly harmed or at risk.

CHAPTER 3

Charting Your Own Course

"The most important rule is to formulate, clearly and precisely, the goal to be reached, and then to retain it unswervingly in mind throughout all the stages of execution, which are often long and complex."

—ROBERTO ASSAGIOLI

What We Believe

We each have a belief system, a context within which we understand ourselves and the world around us. It forms early. The traumas and dramas, large and small, that we experience in early childhood influence what we come to trust to be true and how we behave, feel, and think throughout our lives.

The problem is that these belief systems are largely formed unconsciously and aren't tested until a Big Trauma, like a violent occurrence you might have witnessed or experienced yourself, occurs. Our support systems often collapse or don't support us when we need them most. What we once thought was true turns out not to be.

Consciously and purposefully taking the time to examine your life experiences and core attitudes and values can help you overcome current issues you may be facing. Looking inward, you may uncover unhealed trauma and dysfunction that could be impacting your thinking and well-being in ways that are more harmful than helpful to you. In so doing, the path ahead may be clearer than it is now or may change in some significant, positive way because of your openness to self-discovery.

What we don't know about the impact of trauma on every element of our psyches can hurt and control us in unseen ways. What we misunderstand or misinterpret about ourselves, others, and the world around us can lead us down paths that may not be of our own design or move us toward self-destructive behaviors.

We are often steered astray by the lies we tell ourselves and come to believe are true. They become part of the foundation upon which we build our lives and relationships. We do this largely through a process of adaptation based upon the beliefs of those around us and grounded in our own early experiences.

For example, in my life, the love I was given was what I came to believe love was. When my father loved me, I felt safe. When he rejected me, I felt confused and empty. I felt abandoned by the person I trusted and needed most in the world.

Our relationship was filled with contradictions. I couldn't blame Dad or conclude that his love was flawed in some way. I figured it must be me, even though I had no evidence that was true. That's what I believed, and I became someone who went to great lengths to avoid losing love once I gained it.

What if the family dynamics and pains you were born into didn't start with you, your siblings, or your parents? What if they were predetermined and predestined by the generations of your family that came before all of you? What if you are living within a belief system and took on a role that no longer serves you as an adult? Or, maybe in retrospect, it never did.

The major traumatic event, compounded by those early events in my life, led me to reexamine everything I had come to believe. The tenderness and compassion I found with my wonderful partner and confidant, Norm, in the months following Dad's death gave me renewed faith in humankind and myself.

My graduate studies after Dad's death and my work with people formed the basis of my new understanding of who I am, how I behave, think, and feel, and why. Looking back, I wish the desperate fight to survive had not been the impetus for my self-exploration, but it was.

I visualize helping you proactively face your struggles, hardships, and dilemmas, not solely out of urgent necessity but because you chose to. I share your challenges and celebrate your efforts to do the hard work of replacing destructive patterns with more current, relevant, and trustworthy knowledge as you discover those elements for yourself.

A Framework for Healing Trauma

After Dad's death, I began my journey without a roadmap, wandering the desert that my life had abruptly become. I was searching for understanding and comfort. I urgently needed a sanctuary to recuperate and find my way. I set out to find a place to escape the darkness that surrounded me.

I had to build a new belief system when my old one failed me. Looking at my life with new eyes, I gradually gained insight into myself, how I behave, and the roles I played in my family. I came to recognize the self-destructive ways I used to block my path to a healthy self-image, success, and unconditional love.

I evaluated my strengths and weaknesses and realized I was much smarter than my family had been willing to acknowledge. My teachers and professors placed me at the top of my class or very near the top. When others in my courses were questioning their understanding of complex psychological theory, I found I often had an instant understanding of the teaching being offered. Recognizing these qualities profoundly changed my self-image.

At times along the way I wanted to close my mind when what I needed most was to keep it open. When I felt weary and overly emotional from the pressures of being a full-time student and mother, I became active in positive things that I knew I could do, like growing vegetables, raising roses, cheering for my son at his soccer games, and cooking for gatherings of family and friends.

In my new reality, I accepted responsibility for myself and the unintended interpersonal consequences that are part of change. I found great improvements in many of my relationships and ended or reshaped others that were not healthy. I learned how to be forgiving of others and myself.

The power of the journey is reflected in its outcomes. I found lost parts of myself, truths I had hidden, feelings I had rejected. I discovered a brave new world that I feel more at home in and a me that is reflective of my deepest and most true nature.

That same opportunity exists for you. The road ahead can be filled with new understanding and insight into what drives you under the surface so that you can make the unconscious, conscious. The healing journey offers the prospect of foregoing judgment on self and others. It's not an easy road or a straight path, but it is worth it in the end, as we loosen the grip that past and present challenges often have over us.

In psychology, there is a truism that you can't change what you don't know needs to be different. There is also an understanding in the therapeutic world that you either deal with the problem your client is facing or you deal with their resistance to dealing with the problem. One way or another, getting to the underlying problem and finding a resolution is the surest path to peace of mind and fulfilled aspirations.

The research and theories that I have included in this book are intended to explain some of the many mysteries of being human. The practices and suggestions provided can give you the tools for change. The questions asked will, I hope, get you thinking in new ways.

In the process, you will be encouraged to expand your tolerance for truth and minimize the negative impact of trauma. You will be helped to move beyond your fears. You will find support and kinship in these pages as you refuse to settle for less than you deserve and learn to cherish alone time while improving the quality of your relationships with others.

You will also be challenged to explore how the victim-perpetrator cycle that often results from trauma can be broken, and you'll be aided in finding a healthy way out of dysfunctional patterns of thinking and being.

You can learn to stop retraumatizing yourself and access your healthy psyche. In rethinking where you are now, you may be better able to determine where you want to go, what problems you want to resolve, and what changes you want to make.

Utilize the circumstances of your life right now to motivate yourself to change. Dig deeply within, strengthen your resolve, and unbury truths long hidden in dark corners that you have avoided until now. The power to create change is within you.

You deserve the best out of this life, and these are stressful times we live in—physiologically, psychologically, and emotionally. We each crave feelings of safety and security. What better time than now to set out on a journey of discovery and renewal?

PART II

Drama and Trauma

CHAPTER 4

Beyond Our Control

"Watch the stars.
We can only see so far.
Someday, you'll know where you are."

—THE ALAN PARSONS PROJECT, *DAYS ARE NUMBERS*

IT'S IMPORTANT THAT WE COME TO UNDERSTAND, FIRST theoretically and then personally, the many ways trauma impacts and leaves its imprint on us—body, mind, and spirit. What I know now as I write this book would have been of great comfort to me when I lost my father and had to come to grips with family dysfunction.

It wasn't, however, until much later that I was introduced to the work of Professor Franz Ruppert, PhD, and his pioneering theories and practices in the field of Psychotraumatology, the study of our psychological responses to trauma. Dr. Ruppert has focused his work on the ways in which trauma, from early childhood on, impacts us in seen and unseen ways, at every level of our being.

His work has been extremely valuable in my own healing and my work with others. I want to make it accessible to you here. You never know when you may need a roadmap to deeper understanding.

Dr. Ruppert discusses the three basic mental states that we might find ourselves in relative to our circumstances and experiences: healthy, surviving, or traumatized. To be in a healthy state, he explains, we must feel safe, and when we do, we have a sense of inner calm and contentment. This part of the psyche maintains its hold on reality and is able to self-regulate. We are able to seek resolution for whatever conflict may arise.

In the traumatized psyche, we suffer from the agonizing feelings that the trauma awakened in us, such as fear, pain, anger, despair, and shame. In the survival mindset, argues Dr. Ruppert, we search for escape strategies. The unbearably stressful events we have suffered take a backseat to lifesaving action that serves to numb the thoughts and feelings triggered by the traumatic event and held in the traumatized mind. Whatever tactics we use for survival have a deep and long-lasting impact on our actions later in life, even when no trauma threatens us.

Here is a visual depiction of this split that occurs in the mind, according to Dr. Ruppert.

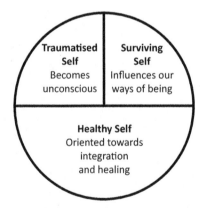

The human psyche split through Psychotrauma
— Franz Ruppert,
Who Am I in a Traumatised and Traumatising Society

It may help to deepen your understanding of the psychological impact of trauma on your life if you take a few minutes to think back to a time when you underwent a trauma, big or small. What were you thinking? How did you feel? When you were at your lowest point, did you know somewhere in you that there could be a safe place to fall? What steps did you take that allowed you to find safety and solace? Or have you?

States of Mind

If we feel unsafe or if our sense of well-being is threatened, we become stressed, and our perceptions and feelings change. We become, out of necessity, focused on the danger or threat we face, whatever it might be. Our thoughts, feelings, and actions can become aggressive in an effort to fight off the danger and survive the threat. We become our traumatized self, searching for survival strategies or frozen in fear.

Trauma becomes the sole occupant of the mind for a time. The shocking and devastating event you have endured or the ongoing, repeated suffering you experienced in your community, home, intimate relationship, workplace, or school—or the collision of both—are all-consuming. You no longer know what it means to be in a safe and healthy frame of mind. You don't know who to trust. You don't know what to do. Fear dominates your thinking.

At other times, under great stress, we become so frightened that we flee or become immobilized and are unable to act at all. Like a possum playing dead under threat, we go into shock. Our heart rate and breathing slow. Our bodies stiffen. We don't dare move. We just want to survive, and we look for ways to do that. It isn't until the threat has been neutralized that we can return to a healthy state of mind, begin to relax, and feel safe again.

From my own experience, I was in a traumatized state from the moment I first learned of Dad's deadly encounter; The rest of my mind and psyche were temporarily unavailable to me. What I know is that I couldn't cope, and any actions I sought to take to relieve the stress failed to save or comfort me. My stress levels soared, making the situation worse.

It is in this state that we fall into full trauma mode. It is a form of going unconscious that allows us to hide from and escape the threatening circumstances we find ourselves in as much as possible. Psychologically, we split off from or disassociate from our trauma. It is, in essence, our psyche protecting us from the horror or disbelief we are experiencing.

While in this state, we may be protecting ourselves from our suffering for a time as we fight to adjust to a reality that has been seriously altered. We aren't able to think clearly or act rationally. We are weakened. Movement seems labored. We become physically and emotionally numb, or the sense of loss and grief we feel is almost overwhelming.

In my case, my loss basically outstripped my psychological ability to cope for a time. Nothing I had learned or experienced prior could have prepared me. I came to understand, amid this drama, that the dysfunction in my family and the isolation I felt only served to undermine my ability to stabilize or feel safe when I most needed to. In my mind, I had nowhere to turn—no one who could bring me comfort.

The days that followed my father's murder are hard to describe.

There was a large funeral at Temple Emanu-El in the main synagogue, a few blocks from our home. I learned later that there were over a thousand people in attendance, but shock kept me from seeing anyone in particular or hearing their words.

To me, it was a blur—just something, one more thing, I had to get through. Dad, I thought in the early days, was the lucky one. He was at peace. He was free. He didn't have to face any of this. In those days and forevermore, I lost the fear of dying. Instead, I feared more the truth of what my life had become.

I remember walking up the hill from Temple to our family home on Clay Street, where the nightmare started mere days before. Reporters and police were everywhere. The media could not leave the story alone and sensationalized it at a time that should have been held sacred, at least for a few days.

The house was overflowing with well-meaning and caring people, stunned and scared that something like this could happen again. I found little comfort in the gathering. Emotionally, I was unreachable and, therefore, irreconcilable. Even those who loved me and were close by couldn't comfort me. I was unable to receive their love in any way that would significantly resolve my loss.

All I could think to do was to escape the house and drive to Baker's Beach in the Presidio, where I hoped I would find some solace in what had always been one of my safe places. I parked in the empty lot at the entrance, took off my shoes and stockings, and walked barefoot to the water's edge. The beach was empty, and visibility was limited by a grey November mist. I burrowed my toes into the cold sand as I had done since Dad first introduced me to this beach.

I drew deep breaths of the cool and salty air that mingled with the salty tears now streaming down my face.

In a way, I welcomed this solitude because I knew that my state of mind was different than it had ever been before. I felt like shrieking, and I did. I felt like crying out loud, and I did. I looked for the horizon that was lost in the fog. I felt so angry that I began stamping my feet in the shallow water.

I was thinking about the person who pulled the trigger and wondered how in God's name anyone could ever do that to another human being. I screamed out, "Dad, where did you go? How can I get you back?" The only answers I received were the deep tones of the foghorns and the sound of the water racing across the sand.

I looked up the steep cliffs to the house once owned by my grandparents. The warm light glowing in the sunroom reminded me of the many days I spent there with my Grandpa Garrett, waiting for Dad to pick me up after work. But now, they were both dead and I was alone on the beach.

Those were indeed my darkest hours. That night, however, I had no idea where I was or whether I would find myself. How could I ever understand the violence that had altered my world forevermore or accept man's inhumanity to man? Was there any part of my mind that had been spared this devastating blow? At that moment, that was a question for which I had no answer.

Facing an Altered Reality

At times like I just described, it seems difficult to imagine we can reclaim our healthy mind and feel safe again. My own experience taught me that and was reinforced by many client experiences I've had over the years.

I often think back to one client, Marie, whom I worked with years ago and whose violent husband, Joel, was threatening her where she worked. My organization, Confidante, was called in to mitigate the danger. She had finally found the courage to file for divorce and seek a protective order. Joel threatened her livelihood, her life, and the well-being of their children and her coworkers.

It was a terrible ordeal that ended with his suicide outside the home they once shared with their three children. Marie and the kids tried to reason with him that night, but in the end, he shot himself as they watched in horror.

Talking to Marie the following night, in my mind I questioned whether she would ever feel safe again. I wondered if she would somehow blame herself for his death. I remember her saying to me, "If I just stayed with him, he'd be alive." I reassured her that she'd done what she needed to do to save herself and her children. "You chose survival," I insisted. "For his own reasons, he did not. It was too late for him but not for you and the kids."

Marie's only motive for leaving her marriage was to end the years of domestic violence she had suffered through. It took her a long time, but in the end, she was able to act in her and her children's best interests. She wanted to protect her children from the same type of abuse she had endured in her youth, at the hands of her father. Instead, with her marriage to Joel, she had placed herself and her children in the same danger she had suffered.

Finally, after 15 years, she exited the fog of the traumatized psyche. She put her survival strategy into action, unfortunately with tragic results. I knew it would be a long time before Marie's traumatized self would find peace, but fortunately, she did have a strong support system with family, friends, and coworkers who rushed to her side.

I've lost touch with Marie over the years, but I can only pray she found a safe place to fall and is living a healthier life. I hope she has successfully broken the chain of abuse that haunted her life and led her into unhealthy relationships. I hope she has learned to laugh again and can sleep soundly at night, unafraid.

It's worth noting that the younger we are when we experience traumatic circumstances, the easier it is for us to be drawn into relationships that are self-injurious and unhealthy as we get older, as Marie was. In this way, trauma can pass from generation to generation.

The opposite can also occur. Trauma can turn us into aggressors. Individuals, for example, who have undergone childhood physical or sexual abuse can become perpetrators of abuse in later relationships. Once the cycle begins, it is difficult to break and often ends in more tragedy. Trauma has the power to drive our choices in unseen ways that can result in repeated reinjury, keeping the original pain active in our lives.

The longer we live in the shadow of trauma, the more difficult it becomes to recover our healthy selves. It feels as though there is no escape from this vicious cycle. We are either striking out or being hurt. We are either suffering alone or in relationships that aren't safe. We are alive but we aren't living.

Recovering our healthy psyche is a struggle we can never give up on. Our survival instincts propel us to escape the trauma we have experienced. The journey is hard but healing. Safety is the destination and a healthy psyche is the reward. We can once again enjoy the many pleasures life has to offer.

Dr. Ruppert describes the splitting of the psyche when we suffer trauma. He also assures us that our survival strategies are lifesaving in grave situations and have a great influence on us later in life. It's true, too, that even when there is no longer an immediate threat, our psychological structures continue to function as if we are in mortal danger. At the same time, it's also true that the healthy part of our psyche remains and continues to grasp reality, manage, and regulate itself. It also preserves for us our sense of inner calm and safety.

As I came to understand our individual vulnerability to danger and threats, I realized that I had been clinging to what was only the illusion of safety. I didn't really feel safe growing up. I underestimated how deeply the dysfunctional circumstances of my youth undermined my ability to confront the trauma of Dad's death. Healthy instincts eluded me.

The lack of bonding with my mother as a child created a devastating lack of comfort and care at the time we were both suffering the grief of Dad's death and Mom's trauma as a witness to it. I realized then that my sense of safety came from my father and now he was gone.

It took me a full year to come out of the shocking state of mind I found myself in. I knew I needed to pick up the pieces of my life and rearrange them around the reality that Dad was no longer part of my day-to-day world. He wasn't at the office on 50 Francisco Street where we'd worked together.

Dad wasn't gazing out at the San Francisco Bay on a clear day or resting on the couch under the grey-green plaid blanket that is now in my house. I couldn't escape the violence that took him away and changed my life forever. But how I let violence change me was in my hands, and for the first time in years, I was formulating a plan. I had a sense of direction I'd been missing for a long time.

The passage of time helped. The shock started to wear off. My children needed me. Grief therapy with a compassionate counselor was invaluable. My deepening friendship with Norm, and his sage legal counsel, helped me discover a path forward.

I couldn't stay in my father's company and run it for my family, Norm told me one day. He was right and I knew it. With his help, I found a buyer and sold the insurance business. I no longer looked for Dad's car in the parking garage or sat in his chair behind his desk in his office or lived the life I had when he was a vital part of it.

I studied the healing work of Psychosynthesis, the brainchild of Dr. Roberto Assagioli, and found self-understanding and peace of mind. I read the beautiful prophetic works of the Catholic theologian Thomas Merton, who gave me faith when my own religious beliefs failed to support me.

All of these and more actions helped me to discover my healthy psyche. I went for morning runs again. I began to have fun with my kids, doing the things we all loved to do. Slowly, I moved from survival to a state of mind where I could thrive.

Many changes took place in my now-altered life. My family moved out of San Francisco in 1977. There was no safety to be found there anymore. I entered graduate school. I lost myself in my long-delayed studies in psychology. I reclaimed my dreams.

I was determined to understand a world and human behavior that I no longer did. Perhaps I could find my healthy self again, come to terms with my loss, and understand what it really means to live in a zone of safety within myself and with others. My confidence began to grow as I accomplished things I had long given up on.

When people go through traumatic experiences together, be it in a family, a business, a school, or a community, there is the reasonable expectation or hope that a deeper connection will form and greater understanding will be gained. That didn't happen for me with my family of origin. I wanted to help others who were suffering. I wanted to heal others as I wanted to heal myself so that they, and I, would feel less alone in our sadness and grief.

With Dad gone, the only true connection between my family of origin, the bond that had held us together, melted away. But I knew that I could not focus on what wasn't there or the comfort I didn't have with them. Instead, I turned my attention to finding what I needed where I could succeed in finding it. My choices were more aligned with my own recovery and well-being.

When my mother remarried a year later and embraced her new husband's family, I could understand this was her way of moving on from the trauma that could have defined the rest of her life. Mom had known Bill for most of her adult life. He was her safe place to fall. It seemed natural that these two old friends would find comfort in each other. I remember Mom calling me from Reno to say, "Bill and I just got married. Be happy for me."

"I am," I said, and I was.

Still, at the time, I was angry that Dad could be so quickly replaced in her life, a sentiment that prevented me from embracing Bill. The end result was that I grew more distant from Mom.

I began to adjust to the deep divide that separated us. I didn't want it to be that way, but it was. I didn't seem to be able to alter that reality, though I continued to try, even with my sister. Once, I did invite her out to lunch several years after Dad died. When I asked her if there was anything I could do that would allow us to have some kind of relationship, she said, "No. You had kids and I couldn't. That's unforgivable." I was stunned.

My brother moved to Sacramento and I rarely heard from him or saw him. His wife worked for the state, and he built wooden boats with his own hands. It was, I imagine, his way to survive. On one rare visit, several years later, I remember Garry taking me out to his garage to show me his handiwork after lunch. He was very proud of himself, and he too seemed to be slowly healing.

He turned to me and asked, "Did you ever see Dad change a light bulb?" We laughed. When I said I couldn't remember, Garry's pride in his newfound craft seemed to be his way of compensating for the kind of relationship he had longed for but never had. He finally found something that he was better at than Dad. I felt a deep sadness that my father never had taken an interest in his only son and left him wounded and traumatized.

In the aftermath of trauma, my family scattered like leaves in a cyclone, settling far apart, at least emotionally. With the distance between us, however, I was able to discover myself. My protector was gone, but I was determined to live on in a manner that mattered to me and with the unconditional love, safety, and support I needed. I came to realize that we all react to trauma and loss in our own way and there is no right way to suffer through the grieving process.

Slowly, I was able to move from darkness to a healthier place in my own psyche. I was able to find more inner strength, resilience, and compassion for myself than I knew I had. I wish it hadn't taken this trauma to figure that out, but it did.

If I had an unconditionally loving family to fall back on, I fervently believe it would have greatly eased my suffering. Ultimately, I recovered with the support I had and with the strength of my survival instincts. One thing I learned as I took control of my life again is the value of being gentle and kind with yourself as you seek to recover your healthy state of mind. Remember it's there for you, and you will find it if you don't give up on yourself.

Journaling a Path to Healing

One of the really important things I did is that I began to keep a journal. I wrote my heart out and over the years my journal became a safe place for me to fall and be with myself. I could rage at the world and my family. I could allow myself to feel my emotions in their most raw and irrational state. It was, and is, cathartic and illuminating to me.

Journaling became the gift I gave to myself, and it also deepened the bond I had with Norm. When at times I would read some of my entries to him, they became a powerful tool of understanding and communicating between us. I began to know myself better, and he, too, learned more about me.

I suggest that you find a special notebook or journal to track your thoughts as you embark on this journey with me. You can pick it up at the end of each chapter or whenever you choose. You can capture your thoughts and feelings as you recover parts of yourself that may lie dormant and hidden, awaiting your discovery or self-reflection.

Taking solitary time to contemplate and write can help you to better understand the splits that exist in your own mind. You may find yourself in a healthier state at the end of your writing session than when you began. You will find that it will become easier for you to access your healthy psyche when you are under stress and need it most. It's like exercising a muscle. The more you use it, the stronger and more accessible it becomes.

If you are fortunate and have an unconditionally loving partner or friend, someone who is safe for you, you might consider reading aloud to them from your journal entries. It is a great way to not only deepen a relationship but to also get to know yourself and your loved one better. It is a wonderful way for you to be heard in a world where so many people seem to be more skillful talkers than listeners.

I also encourage you to save your journals in a safe place. You never know when rereading them will spark new understanding. Or, like me, you may use them to refresh your memory if you consider writing a book or sharing your life story with people close to you. My journals have been an invaluable resource to me over the years. They mark the path of stumbles, progress, and evolution.

It's also a great way to better understand the three states of mind discussed in this chapter: the traumatized, the survival, and the healthy psyche so that you can learn to move more freely from an unhealthy state to a healthy one. You will be better able to recognize where you might be stuck and how to get back to a safer and more productive emotional place.

Through journaling, you can make conscious the often-unconscious ways that the impact of past trauma may still be influencing your choices and all levels of well-being and health. By writing and sharing your experiences, you can contribute to your own healing and give voice to parts of you that have suffered in silence.

CHAPTER 5

The Road Back

"Perhaps I am stronger than I think."

—Thomas Merton

ARE YOU ABLE TO RECOGNIZE IN YOUR OWN LIFE THE WAYS TRAUMA
served as a motivator for you to make positive change? Have you led
a more meaningful life than you once did? Did you make healthier
choices in relationships, your work, or your service to others
as a result of some of the hardships you suffered? Are you kinder
to others as a result of the psychological damage done to you by
bullies or abusive figures in your life? It is our drive toward health
and safety, often triggered by trauma, that can lead us to positive
outcomes we might not have sought otherwise. It takes strength
and determination to transform negatives into positives, but the
opportunity always exists in the human spirit to do so.

This is how we can begin to take control of our lives. When we go
through a shattering experience and feel that we have little control
over external events, it is critical to explore ways to shift our perspective to an internal locus of control—one step at a time—where
different possibilities exist.

Among other things, for me, surviving and getting healthy meant
making healthier relationship choices. I kept my distance from
family drama. I embraced those who were not necessarily related by

blood but were related in spirit and provided me with the safe social relationships I craved.

I bonded with my graduate school colleagues who were motivated as much as I was by traumatic occurrences in their lives and the strong desire to help others. My professors and supervisors provided me with guidance and an invaluable education. Norm and I drew closer. I reconnected with long-lost friends. I became less engaged with my family of origin.

As a child, I didn't see that escaping family dysfunction was an option open to me. Now that the choice was mine to make, I didn't want to waste the opportunity I had to nurture myself in ways that I could not have imagined before trauma.

At first, the distancing I sought was a matter of self-preservation and part of my healing. It is how I began to create a safe perimeter around myself and my life. This to me was one of the ways I created a safe place to land and find solace. I started to carve out a new role for myself in a family that was now accentuated by the absence of my father and the devastating nature of his death. I immersed myself in a world foreign to them and nurturing to me.

Human Potential

I studied nonstop for five years. I was living in the heartland of the human potential movement in Marin County in the early 1980s. It was an outgrowth that arose from the counterculture of the 1960s. It focused on cultivating vast capacities that advocates of it believed were largely untapped in most of us.

The prevailing belief was that through the development of human potential we can experience more happiness, creativity, and fulfill-ment. Some of the thought leaders of the movement were names that you might recognize. They included Alan Watts, Victor Frankl, William James, Aldous Huxley, and Carl Rogers, to mention a few.

I know I was hungry for new ways of thinking that had the potential to point me in the direction of a more meaningful life. I exposed myself to each new theorist and spiritual leader who emerged during this time.

I studied heavily in the field of grief and loss, including work with Elizabeth Kubler-Ross and Stephen and Ondrea Levin. I attended meditation retreats with groups of people who had also suffered the emotionally ravaging loss of loved ones. I was humbled to be among them and hear their stories.

I found that in the sharing of our experiences, we are able to disarm the traumas we have suffered. We don't have to use them to reinjure ourselves time after time. We can release their power over us. We learn that we are not as alone as we might think.

In the aftermath of trauma, when we are searching for reasons to move on and make our loss or tragedy mean something, life takes on a heightened sense of urgency. I've worked with many cancer patients over the years and learned valuable lessons from those who have found the tremendous relief and joy of remission. They come to appreciate their lives and health in powerful ways many of us take for granted. Each moment is a gift to be cherished and enjoyed. They want to make every day count. They are able to turn their focus from fearing death to embracing life. They set new goals, bring long-buried dreams to actualization, and embrace those they love with new abandon.

I felt the same commitment to embracing each day. I was on a search for my own healing, and to a large degree, I began to find it. For years, I immersed myself in Psychosynthesis, the brainchild of Dr. Roberto Assagioli, an Italian psychiatrist who survived imprisonment by the fascist regime of Benito Mussolini (definitely one of those Big Traumas). Assagioli was arrested for praying for peace in 1940 and placed in solitary confinement for a month, where he couldn't influence others. Upon his release, he continued his work in hiding, and when World War II ended he returned to Florence and began his legacy work, Psychosynthesis.

A pioneer in the field of humanistic behavior and transpersonal psychology, Assagioli was inspired by Sigmund Freud and Carl Jung. He believed that love, wisdom, creativity, and free will were important components for healthy functioning. Along with Jung, Assagioli helped to validate the spiritual dimension of human nature. He continued to believe in the highest nature of humanity, even though Mussolini's actions were meant to plunge him into the depths of despair.

Who Am I?

My studies of Assagioli's work helped draw me back from a very dark place. His emphasis on the potential of the progressive integration, or synthesis, of the personality and its reorganization around the higher self—the spiritual element of our nature—renewed my faith in myself and the future.

It reinforced the concept that we have a human impulse toward wholeness and healing and that our potential is boundless. Trauma can act like a spark that sets fire to our desire to be our best, live purposeful lives, and bring meaning and hope to the lives of others.

Many of us who have suffered a violent trauma at the hands of another, whether a stranger or a loved one, often suffer a dramatic loss of faith. It's hard at times to know if there is actually a spiritual side of human nature or a higher purpose to our lives. Instead, we come face-to-face with man's inhumanity toward man. It's hard to see the goodness in others when we feel that the goodness in us has somehow been soiled by our experience.

That's in large part why Assagioli's theories on the will and his hopeful approach to psychology can be so helpful. He surely lived as he believed when he found himself imprisoned in solitary confinement. He could have fled toward his traumatized mind, but instead, he found the solace of the healthy psyche.

The trauma he suffered didn't turn him away from what he fervently believed when the intention was to silence him. He decided, by a sheer act of will, how he would spend his time in isolation. He turned that one month into a lifetime of healing work that has helped countless others around the world. Assagioli's theories have sustained the test of time.

I focused on his teachings of free will. I searched for the freedom he spoke of from the emotional, mental, and physical demands of the many subpersonalities that feed the ego and drive our actions. Subpersonalities are psychological formations in our personality that are constructed around basic needs but do not necessarily serve a higher purpose or our best interests.

If you think about the difference between how you act at work as opposed to how you act when you are at home, in social settings, or alone, you will see that these are roles we play. We may, for example, be loving and kind in our interactions with a family member because we have a need to be liked and viewed as trusted. But then, perhaps when we are with other family members who are critical of this person, we join in because, again, we want to be in the know and get satisfaction out of being the purveyor of gossip.

Our actions are often contradictory. These different modes or sub-personalities are activated temporarily to cope with different types of situations or serve our needs in different settings. And in the end, do we really appear trustworthy to anyone? Are we really liked, or do people fear they will become the target of our judgment and criticism, depending upon our needs at any given time?

Another example is of the classic bully in a position of authority in the workplace who misuses his power over subordinates. I'm reminded of a CEO I was retained to coach by his board of directors. During my work with George, he informed me that he enjoyed managing "by intimidation" and that it was the best way to get things done.

That was his way of motivating others to do what he wanted them to do. They feared him, and that satisfied some need in him to be in control and exercise his power. George was not averse to screaming at subordinates or slamming the door in their faces. Those who worked with him saw him as a tyrant, and he seemed not to care. He actually confessed to me that he enjoyed it.

That was his preferred style in the workplace. He took on his bully subpersonality. George told himself: That's the way to get the job done. But when I saw him with his wife at a holiday event, he displayed a totally different persona. George was meek and mild-mannered, himself intimidated by a domineering wife who was even more successful—and unpleasant—than he was. When his wife raised her voice at him and criticized him publicly, he shrank into a corner of the room, where he sullenly nursed a cocktail.

This bully at work cowered at home. George felt powerful at work and powerless in his marriage. The people who worked under him would have wondered who in the world he really was. His wife would have been shocked by his authoritative style at work. These were two subpersonalities of his in different situations, with different needs. But, who was he really? I wondered. Did he even know?

When I confronted George about the disparities I saw in his behavior in these two environments, I asked him to describe how he felt after his wife intimidated him publicly. When I pointed out to him that he evoked the same fear in his subordinates, he told me that neither description reflected who he truly believed himself to be.

As we began to work on these issues, he was able to balance out the needs of his subpersonalities. He understood himself better and was able to positively modify his interactions at home and work. The outcome was an improved, more collegial workplace, a happy board of directors, and a more harmonious relationship with his wife.

These psychological constructs can dominate our personalities and interactions in different situations, but they are not who we truly are. By recognizing these parts, we can better understand ourselves. We can reorganize our personalities around our higher selves and free our will to act appropriately and effectively in any given situation. For me, this process was part of recapturing my power and becoming my authentic self.

There is a simple exercise in Psychosynthesis that I suggest you try when you have some time to yourself. It's called "Who Am I?" and was published in *Synthesis Journal* in 1978. It's still relevant and widely used today.

Find a quiet place, take out a piece of paper or your journal, date it, and then ask yourself the question, "Who am I?" Write down your answer and keep asking yourself the same question over and over again, writing your new answer each time. You will find that you come up with a succession of different answers.

You may find yourself stuck, but keep going. Write as long a list as you like. Give yourself 10 to 15 minutes. By the end, you should have a sense of some of your subpersonalities and the roles you play and identify yourself with in different aspects of your life.

I suggest, too, that you repeat this exercise periodically. The list of who we are and how we are identified at any given time will continue to change. Sometimes we act as if we are our feelings. They dominate our actions. They tell us what's true. At other times, we act as if we are our thoughts. What we think is what's real. We ignore our emotions. Still, at other times, we become identified with the roles we play in our lives. None of these aspects of us are our authentic selves.

Regaining Control

Having the ability to dis-identify from the many parts of ourselves and act upon our highest interest from a spiritual perspective is critical to healing. In the aftermath of trauma, or during the trauma of ongoing dysfunctional circumstances, we need to reassert our free will. If we don't begin to regain control, these elements of human nature whip us around like flags in the wind until we don't know who we are or what we want.

I learned to strive for simplicity and truth in my personal life, supported by a spiritual approach to human behavior and psychology. Assagioli's view that humans are fundamentally healing organisms that suffer temporary malfunctions was inspirational to me.

For example, when I heard myself speaking to my children in ways that were critical and in tones that were harsh, I could see the hurt and confusion on their faces. I couldn't necessarily stop myself at the moment, but I would later step back and ask myself: *Is that you, or is that a part of you that was spoken to in a harsh way when you were young? Is that one of the subpersonalities that formed to defend yourself or is that your essence?*

Perhaps, as Assagioli would surmise, that behavior with my kids was a temporary malfunction that I could recover from. I could be healthier and I could be a more unconditionally loving parent. To know that we are always trying to reestablish harmony and calm at deeper and deeper levels was the reassurance I sought. I put the trauma I had lived through to work and it changed me and my life—for the better.

I hope that you are able to find a place within you that can contain the traumas you have suffered without allowing them to dominate your thinking or control your decisions. We are so much more than the bad things that happen to us or the mistakes we have made. And I firmly believe in our power to change ourselves.

By connecting the impact that trauma has had on your life and holding it in your mind in the ways suggested above, I do believe you will find the impulse and drive toward healing that Dr. Assagioli describes. You will know for certain that there is a higher place within you to look upon the things that have happened to you or others.

CHAPTER 6

Stops Along the Way

"Nothing is more natural than grief, no emotion more common
to our daily experience. It's an innate response to loss in
a world where everything is impermanent."

—STEPHEN LEVINE

IN THE AFTERMATH OF TRAUMA, WHETHER IT INVOLVES SOMEONE'S death, our own near-death experience, an ugly divorce, or facing the truth of family dysfunction, we go through the stages of grief on the path to healing. We have lost someone or something we have relied upon, valued, or loved.

We are altered, often in dramatic ways. We are confronted with the impermanent nature of life. Change, we learn, is the only constant, and sometimes what happens is beyond our control. It's what we do in the face of unexpected change that matters most and is actually within our control.

Once we have accepted that our loss is a reality we can't alter and have gone through denial and isolation, anger, bargaining, depression, and acceptance, we start to look for ways to move onward.

Beyond the first five stages of grief, there is a less-discussed sixth stage. This is our search for meaning, a process that can transmute our loss into a more peaceful understanding and experience. While many people talk about finding closure, it's elusive. I believe finding meaning in our grief is where the true transformative power is.

This is when we begin to let go of what was and never will be again. This is a time when the love we feel for what or who was lost is greater than our grief. This is when we look for ways to move forward, and I hope for you that what's ahead is a more optimistic, healthy, and meaningful path, as has been true in my life.

Above the Rare Bookstore

With my graduate studies complete, I found new meaning when I hung out my first shingle as a counselor and consultant in a rooftop office above a rare bookstore in the quaint city of San Anselmo, California, five minutes from home in 1981. The many book restorers, buyers, and sellers who frequented the bookstore below my office became an important referral source for my new practice.

From my office on the second floor, I could see the San Francisco Theological Seminary and enjoyed the sound of her steeple bell that came to me through the forest. I walked down Shady Lane and visited St. Anselm's Church, whose doors were always open. I would kneel and pray silently. I would light a candle for Dad and share with him what I was learning and doing, tell him how much I missed him, and ask for his advice on current family dramas.

It was a safe, warm, and welcoming environment, everything the city of San Francisco would never be again. Fortunately, too, I discovered that rare book people are quiet, courteous, and friendly, and I found a sense of community. I was changed by my life above the bookstore. I found meaning in helping others. The paradox was that helping to heal others and healing myself turned out to be the same.

Using Psychosynthesis' guided imagery with clients, I sat in wonder and watched as they, with closed eyes, followed my voice. They were transported to traumatic times that they had not been able to face. In my little office above the bookstore, they would confront their demons and journey through fear to the safe haven of their healthy psyches. When they opened their eyes, they seemed more at ease and hopeful. They gained perspective and self-understanding into their experiences.

In my own guided imagery sessions with a grief counselor, I was finally able to confront Dad's killer. In my mind, he was small and not frightening. In my visualization, I was able to overlook the gun that he held in his right hand. My thought was how tragic it was that someone so young was already conditioned to ignore the value of a human life.

Eddie's life didn't matter to his murderer at all. He was just the guy walking down the street with his dog. But somehow, I was able to find a measure of forgiveness and understanding I didn't know I had within me. This process allowed me to modulate my anger for what I began to see as a misguided boy.

I was increasingly able to adjust to the changes that continued to take place in my personal life, including the amicable and mutually agreed upon dissolution of my marriage to Jason in 1982. This was part of moving forward for me.

Jason was a great stepdad to my children. His love for them was a gift of immeasurable value, as was the comfort he provided to us when Dad died. I will always be grateful that he was with me, ran interference with my family, and provided stability for my children when I had nothing to give.

It's true that making major life decisions, such as moving, divorce, or changing professions in the immediate aftermath of trauma or tragedy is not advisable. It can take years, as it did with me, to make significant, well-thought-out changes. But, I believe, for many of us it is important to take stock of our lives when we have been shaken to our core and be able to articulate what we want to be different.

It's important to ask ourselves: Is this relationship or marriage healthy for me? Is the work I am doing meaningful to me? Do I like where I'm living? Do I feel safe? Is there something I've always wanted to do but never have and would regret not doing? Imagine yourself five years from now.

Where do you want to be, what do you want to be doing, and who do you want to be sharing it with? What brings meaning to your life? I know that for me, the trauma I suffered led me down a path to a meaningful life that I could not have foreseen.

Grief and Loss

I could not know that helping others face death would allow me to let go of the grip that Dad's death had on me. In those days, I was still haunted by the thought of him dying alone, depriving us both from sharing a mutual measure of closure. I still feel this burden at times, but it was significantly eased when I had the opportunity to work closely with a patient suffering from terminal cancer.

Her name was Pam and she had been a frequent visitor to the rare bookstore. This case touched me deeply; the treasured art book she gave me on the life and work of famous Spanish architect Antonio Gaudi still sits on the bookshelf in my office.

I watched Pam's health deteriorate over the course of a year when each new round of chemotherapy failed. As death approached, I visited her once or twice a week to offer counsel and comfort. I usually sat in a straight-back chair pulled close to her bed. One particular day that I recall, the sun was warming my back as it came through the curtain-less window of her beautiful home in Marin County's lush rolling hills.

Over time, Pam's bedroom felt more and more like a sick room, less inviting and cozy with each visit. The IV pump hummed as both toxic and nurturing fluids emptied from their respective bags, dripping into the catheter implanted in her sunken chest cavity. A single red rose fought for a place on her small bedside table, crowded with amber pill vials, gauze pads, and glasses of juice and water.

Pam was stretched flat, her small body on the king-sized bed almost lost under the billowing blue down of her comforter. I opened my eyes as I heard her stir, wincing in pain. On this sunlit summer day, just raising her head from the pillow was a strain. The cancer had spread throughout her body, every bone weakened and brittle with the disease. Each movement threatened another break.

"I can't do this anymore," she said softly, close to my ear as I got up to adjust the pillows. I told her I understood.

I had been helping people die for several years in my private practice. But Pam was different; this was more personal. Our families and backgrounds were so similar. We didn't know each other, but we could have. We were the same age. We grew up within 20 minutes of each other and our families were both members of Temple Emanuel.

Her son and mine were the same age. It could have been my boy losing me. I could picture myself feeling what she felt, knowing I was about to die, but I could not imagine suffering as bravely as she did.

When she spoke, I moved closer to her so that I could hear her weakened voice. "I hurt everywhere," she said. "I don't want to live. Not like this. Not anymore."

She closed her eyes against the pain. I placed one hand gently on her hand, careful not to put any pressure on it. With my other hand, I moved my chair slightly to the left so that the sun could shine on her where she lay.

When Pam opened her eyes again and looked at me, she said, "Help me say goodbye. Please. Help my son understand how much I love him; tell him that I'm sorry I have to leave him. Talk to my family. Make them see I need to go. I'm ready."

"I'll do my best," I said.

"Promise you will be with me when I die," her voice barely above a whisper.

I promised I would.

At that moment, I came to understand the relationship between unconditional love and healing. I knew from my own experience that I had found meaning in my loss, and that awareness allowed me to help Pam and her family. Although I could not heal Pam's body, perhaps I could help heal her spirit by giving her a loving send-off from life.

In the end, she would not be alone. Our time that day ended but not before she had turned her face from the sunlight and drifted off again. I whispered, "Goodbye," but she didn't hear me. I am grateful to report that it was not my last visit.

A few weeks later, I was able to keep my promise. I was there with Pam when she passed. That final day, I brought with me a strawberry milkshake as we agreed I would. She took her last sip and within an hour, she faded, one labored breath at a time until there were no more.

Pam's death and my father's murder are actual losses that had occurred. As part of the grieving process, the final steps of acceptance and the search for meaning allowed me to make their deaths and lives matter.

Pandemics Past and Present

Given we are in the midst of an overwhelming pandemic as I write, I am reminded of another pandemic, one that I found myself amid in the 1980s. To further illuminate how collective traumas can impact us, I want to share my memories of the HIV/AIDS crisis when I was in the early days of my career.

At that point in time, Norm and I had known each other for nearly 10 years. With each year, our bond grew stronger. When he asked me to join his young company in the fight to stem the spread of this terrible disease, I couldn't say no. This turned out to be the next step in my journey and an opportunity for us to work closely together.

In 1985, Norm had cofounded Lifesource, a company that became one of the premier regional providers of home infusion therapy in the U.S.

The company pioneered cancer chemotherapy and home infusion protocols for antibiotic therapies, pain control, and intravenous nutrition. They also pioneered the first HIV/AIDS home therapy, support programs, nutrition, and wound care at the height of the terrible epidemic that spread through the Bay Area. They received a humanitarian award for their efforts.

In 1986, Norm called me one afternoon and asked if he could stop by and see me. He told me that one of the Lifesource nurses came back to the office after treating an AIDS patient several nights before and was hysterical. "It took me three hours to calm her down. She was removing the oxygen tubes to clean them and part of his nose came off with them," Norm said.

He continued, "It's this Kaposi's sarcoma, an AIDS-defining cancer, and the infections that are ravaging their bodies. Nobody knows how to treat it. We are using every chemo regimen and antibiotic in the books. None of it is working."

We agreed that I would need a small office where Norm and the nurses could have access to me 24/7. Over the next month, I transitioned my existing clients to a colleague from graduate school and turned my attention full-time to the nurses, where I became Lifesource's first Director of Psychosocial and Human Resources Services. My work there was eye-opening from the first day.

So many young men were struck so quickly with the deadly sickness that seemed to target the gay community. The Castro District in San Francisco that had gained renown for its culture of open expressions of homosexuality was particularly hard hit.

Death, dying, and grieving for lost loved ones became part of daily life during the AIDS pandemic and was a nightmare for the medical community battling to save lives and find answers. There were so many unknowns associated with the disease. People were afraid to use public toilets or shake hands.

Nurses in hospitals refused to bring meals to AIDS patients. Doctors debated whether or not they had a moral obligation to treat people with AIDS. The medical community was at a loss for how to treat the disease. Lifesource nurses and doctors of pharmacology were on the front lines of the battle, fighting for the lives of their patients.

Lifesource and other health professionals faced serious safety concerns. Just about every nurse that was accidentally pricked with a needle got it too. In addition to the challenges Norm's team faced treating the victims of this deadly pandemic, they had to also establish new protocols to dispose of needles safely so that their nurses didn't suffer the same fate.

It was intense in the early days. Other people's trauma had my full attention. The meaningful life I had been yearning for came in a way I could not have imagined. The magnitude of it was almost overwhelming, but the fulfillment I felt was worth any sacrifice. I invited the nurses to call me anytime if they thought I could provide them some help.

I accompanied them on home visits with AIDS patients as well as our patients on cancer chemotherapy treatments. I debriefed them when we returned to the office. I sat in on the daily clinical meetings and led them in brief guided imagery sessions to start the day. It was a challenge to stay on top of their feelings as they were being retraumatized daily.

I saw true professionals risking their own lives to help and comfort others in a battle that felt like we were losing, and I was their safe place to fall. At the end of their long and trying days, they could let down their guard, release their feelings, tell their stories of horror, and find the strength to face the next day and the next.

It was draining work but it was also the most worthwhile effort of my life up to that point. By the time I had been there for a year, I had them better prepared emotionally. I had convinced them they were indeed the most important people in the lives of patients and loved ones and that I hoped their contributions to the suffering of others was rewarding to them.

I felt the power of unconditional love that brought these brave, compassionate people to their chosen profession and the aid of those in desperate need. Norm and I were working side by side and I couldn't imagine myself with a better partner or working toward a more worthwhile goal.

We would walk away at the end of a long day, exhausted but gratified by the progress we were making. I was grateful for the opportunity to give back to this man who had already given me so much over the years since Dad died, and we grew close. We had, in each other, a safe place to fall and let go of the trauma we witnessed every day. We were able to recover enough at the end of one day to face the next day and the next.

My work at Lifesource was both rewarding and demanding, certainly testing my emotional fortitude and professional acumen. I was challenged every day with the painful pleas of terminally ill patients begging me to talk to their families and convince them to let go, to say goodbye, and let them die.

It was gut-wrenching, each story a human tragedy. When I was asked by a patient to help her loved ones let go because she was ready to go, I did my best to help them understand that the quality of her life had deteriorated to a point that she didn't want to suffer anymore. Finally, they understood that what they wanted was not what she wanted. In the end, with hospice there, they had their chance to say their goodbyes and she peacefully let go of her life.

Helping others die—and watching others die—is traumatic, but never getting to say goodbye to a loved one can be tragic. In fact, "I didn't get to say goodbye" has become a headline I see more and more frequently as the deaths from COVID-19 continue to mount locally, nationally, and worldwide. How many times have I said that about Dad? It's something you never get over.

You lose the chance to say a proper goodbye or talk about your life with a loved one. You don't get the chance to tell them how much they meant to you when someone you love is suddenly wrenched away from you. With dying patients ravaged by AIDS, their devastated loved ones, and caregivers, I did what I could to help them say farewell.

With Pam, I was there throughout the last painful year of her life and at the moment of her death. We spoke a great deal about getting closure and what that would look like for her. During her painful decline, she asked that I seek the help of a videographer who would come to the house. We would film her as she spoke to her family, sharing with them how she wanted to be remembered, what they each meant to her, and what she dreamed of for them in their lives after her death.

This was Pam's way of getting closure and giving closure to her loved ones who were struggling to accept that her traumatic loss was inevitable and fast approaching. It was a beautiful experience to be part of, and when the time came, her family was so grateful that she had given them this gift, even as they mourned her loss.

Years after Pam's death and my work with Lifesource, I was inspired to conduct a weekend retreat with a minister friend of mine at a mediation center in Mendocino County. The workshop was titled "Writing Your Own Eulogy" and was as powerful as any workshop I had ever conducted.

This chapter has focused on death and dying and the power of finding meaning in the losses we suffer. While it may seem like a strange suggestion to make, I ask that you think about your own mortality. What and who has brought meaning to your life over the years? I encourage you to reflect upon what you would like to be remembered for and what you would want those you love to know about what they meant to you. If you could write your own eulogy, what would you want to say? Is your story all that you would want it to be at the end of your life? Would you be able to say you have no regrets?

At the workshop, each participant read their eulogy aloud to the group. It was a brave thing to do. There were no dry eyes in the room. People were able to discuss what they might change about their lives, what they regretted. Before we ended that day, I asked the participants what they want to be able to write and say at the end of their days that wasn't part of their eulogy that day.

Think about that for yourself. It might point you in unexpected directions or motivate you to reach out to someone you have lost touch with but still cherish. I'd like to think that in this present moment, it's not too late to make meaningful change or bring new meaning to the losses we have suffered and to the rest of our lives.

CHAPTER 7

The Power of Unconditional Love

*"Love is our true destiny. We do not find the meaning of life
by ourselves alone—we find it with another."*

—THOMAS MERTON

LET'S TALK ABOUT LOVE. WE HAVE SPOKEN OF GRIEF AND LOSS, BUT I
believe it's critical that each of us understands the difference between
unconditional love and conditional love so that we can apply this
knowledge to our own experiences.

Let me begin by describing for you what I mean when I speak of
unconditional love and its extraordinary ability to heal when we are
in the midst of, or the aftermath of, trauma. It is unchanging and
consistent. It is forgiving and accepting. We feel safe in its presence.
We find comfort in its arms.

Conditional love, on the other hand, is what my experience of love
had been growing up. It is love that has to be "earned." It can be
taken away without warning. There are demands that come with it
that may be consciously or unconsciously set. Nobody tells us those
expectations are there so that we can do our best to avoid them or at
least be prepared when we run into them.

Often, we don't know that they existed or that we haven't met those
conditions until that love is withdrawn. When we love someone
conditionally, we often want them to look, act, think, or feel in ways

that fit our expectations or we will feel justified in withholding our love from them. It, generally, is not a safe place to fall but it may be the only kind of love we've known.

Unconditional Love

My introduction to unconditional love came when I least expected it but needed it most. Norm helped me find meaning when I had lost it. I know I could not have found the solace, safety, and strength I did without him.

It's ironic to think that Dad had introduced Norm and me two months before he died. One morning, the three of us found ourselves in the hallway that separated Norm's law office from our insurance office. We exchanged pleasantries, spoke briefly, and then we all went back to work. Norm, Dad told me, was a good guy who did legal work for him. Other than that, he didn't say too much.

When I really got to know Norm, he already seemed to understand the closeness of my relationship with Dad. I knew I had been a topic of discussion between them. He knew what Dad's life and loss meant to me in ways I never expected. Just when I was feeling most alone, I found new hope in a kindred spirit.

My trust in my fellow man began to slowly return as I grew close to Norm. He became a constant source of strength, encouragement, and love in my life. I felt understood and safe again in a world that had become dangerous and frightening overnight.

One day in particular stands out in my mind. I was in Norm's office to sign some documents he had prepared for me, finalizing the sale of Dad's business. When I handed the signed contract over to him and he reached out to take it from me, I saw the look of understanding on his face, a compassion I had been searching for. He suggested that we walk across the Embarcadero to The Crow's Nest Restaurant, a favorite of locals and tourists.

I recalled hearing from a mutual friend who knew both of us that Norm had lost his father in an accident years before and still mourned him. I welcomed the opportunity to share memories and grieve together.

"Let's grab the red umbrella over there on the deck," he said, and we sat down opposite one another. He took off his tie, unbuttoned the cuffs of his shirt, and rolled up the sleeves. "No more business," he said, "Just two friends getting to know each other better." I was happy to be spending more personal, private time with him away from the office.

"Since your dad's gone I can tell you this," he said. "You were the light of his life. You were the only person in your family that he trusted. He wanted to protect you."

"That's comforting to know," I said.

We enjoyed our lunch in peace. It's always been important to me to feel comfortable in silence with someone close, as I did now. That's a mark of safety in a relationship. You don't have to talk to feel seen, heard, and understood. You feel comfort in their presence.

I looked across the table at Norm, who had closed his clear green eyes and moved his chair closer to mine to feel the sun on his back. At that moment, I was struck by how handsome he was. There was no mistaking his Viking heritage or inner strength.

I had been under so much stress that I hadn't even noticed before. Now that he had eased my anxiety and tension, I was seeing things with more detail and listening and hearing more. It seemed that my respirations and heartbeats had slowed, and I was feeling content.

As we finished our lunch, I broached the subject of his father's death. When I saw him close his eyes, hesitate, and begin to breathe deeply, I almost regretted asking. When he steadied himself and opened his eyes, he said, "Telling you how I survived my dad's death might help you a little."

He warned me that he still couldn't talk about his father without shedding tears because, he said, "Nobody could have loved their dad more than I loved mine."

I thought to protest but instead said, "I think hearing about how you survived would be a meaningful thing for me too. My tears have all but dried up."

"Don't worry," he said, "they'll be back." I hoped he was right.

Norm began by sharing with me that his greater family is closer than any family he's ever known. He said, "The love in my family was probably deepened by the ending of the Second World War when my uncles returned home."

I remember Norm's description of the big house he grew up in, always filled with laughter and music that sat on a country road in Bakersfield. "Our house was a healing place for the uncles who felt the effects of combat. They suffered from what they called 'shell shock' in those days, long before it was called PTSD."

"I think what made us different was my father's ability to be a catalyst for unconditional love between the rest of us," he explained. "Everyone loved my dad. He was like a magnet of acceptance, caring, and love, and he was not afraid to say it. He was definitely a healer in the first degree. He made everything fun," Norm said.

Holidays at his house were family affairs looked forward to by all. Preparation in their Bakersfield home included family members coming to work in the huge family vegetable garden, picking fruits, nuts, and vegetables, and then cooking together. I couldn't help but compare Norm's family experiences with my own. Only one of my uncles was in the war. I was too young to remember his return, and the talk about the war in our family was of the plight of our ancestors and the deaths of six million Jews.

Sometimes we did have big holiday parties when Dad's siblings and my cousins came to the house, but the ambiance wasn't as Norm described. We didn't do much cooking together and we bought our fruits and vegetables at the market. Hired help did most of the holiday preparation and cooking in the kitchen. "Life in Bakersfield sounds pretty great," I said. "I can only imagine how your dad was missed."

Norm told me that his father was killed while he was living in San Francisco attending law school. Norm had pulled an all-nighter in the library preparing for exams and didn't come home until dawn the following morning. When he opened the door of his apartment, the living room was full of uncles.

At first, he was thrilled and hoped maybe they were there to kidnap him and take him deep-sea fishing in the bay. But when he saw the looks on their faces, that thought disappeared. It was at this point in the story that Norm hesitated. He looked down and went silent for a moment as the tears he'd promised began streaking his face.

"My five uncles surrounded me," Norm continued. "And then Uncle John said, 'Norm, we have some terrible news. Earlier yesterday afternoon your dad was killed in a head-on collision on the causeway bridge near Yuba City. He died instantly. We couldn't reach you. We've been waiting for you all night.'"

As Norm's knees collapsed under him, he said, "Ten hands pulled me into a circle of loving support that kept me from falling." I now had a real-life example of what it means, literally, to have a safe place to fall into unconditional love.

At that moment, I knew I shared a deeper kinship with Norm, which I experienced as sweet solace. I thought back on how many people had approached me with solemn faces and words like, "my thoughts and prayers are with you" or "I know how you feel," which gave me little comfort.

In contrast, Norm's words relieved my feeling of isolation. Now there was one other human being in my realm; I was no longer totally alone. His tears were remarkable to me. I strained to remember a time I saw Dad cry, but none came to mind.

Norm went on to tell me that his uncles took him home to the healing place that had just lost its founder. He recounted that there were 14 family members gathered when they reached the house and that all were feeling the same loss. "They surrounded Mom, Sis, and me in a group hug," Norm told me, "the kind Dad would have organized if he was there. All these blue eyes, filled with sorrow and love, looked back at me. I wasn't alone with my grief."

Norm's extended family gathered for his father's funeral several days after his accident. They went back to the house after the service and barbequed steaks just like his father would have done if one of them had died. Norm said, "I lost count of how many hugs we had that day. I just remember being in the middle of all of my family and the love that flowed between and around us."

I found myself crying for both of us. My tears hadn't dried up as I feared they had. I received my first handkerchief from Norm that day (and over the years, I have accumulated many more). My tears and I had found a safe place to fall.

I recalled the awkward, tentative hugs I received from family members after we learned of Dad's death that led me to flee to Baker's Beach for the comfort and solace I couldn't find with them. I remembered wrapping my arms around myself as I stood shivering, alone on the beach. "I would have given anything to be in the center of one of those hugs after Dad died," I said.

"My family would have gladly accepted you and mourned for you," Norm said and touched the back of my hand gently.

What Norm had just described is the kind of love I dreamed of, and he had it from the time he was born. When his father died, he learned just how important that love was.

Unconditional love is a uniting force shared in good times and bad—healing when we hurt, comforting when we're scared, given and received without hesitation or expectation. It never disappoints or disappears.

I would ask you: When you lost someone dear or found yourself in need of loving arms to hold you up, were they there? When you recall your childhood, would you say you grew up in an unconditionally loving home, and if so, did you pass that same kind of love on to your children?

Or, did you inherit conditional love that was passed on through the generations, from your grandparents to your parents, and then to you? How has that conditional love impacted your life and shaped the love you have to give?

I fervently believe, from the bottom of my heart, that each of us is deserving of the kind of unconditional love I talk about in this chapter and others. The more we each learn of the nature of this quality of love—how to give it and how to receive it—the better able we will be to break the cycles of inherited trauma and feel the comfort we have the capacity to provide to each other.

Love Unlike My Own

That day was a turning point for me. Hope returned. Old dreams resurfaced. The prospect of starting over did not seem so bleak anymore. And I had a new understanding forming about the nature and power of unconditional love. I will never underestimate its healing power.

As I learned to receive it, I gradually learned to accept it and give it back. I no longer felt limited by the love I had learned in my family, the kind that came with strings attached. Within the arms of unconditional love, I found the comfort and acceptance I had longed for. I learned of its nonjudgmental nature that allowed me to grow and change. I discovered the true power of forgiveness. I was able to move through life with new confidence.

Norm had many more examples of how his family experiences provided him guidance on ways to make interactions with others harmonious. To me, he's the master of safe places. He made me laugh and he made me tear up with his stories. The emotional connection between us was undeniable.

I knew there would be rough days ahead for me, adjusting to the world without Dad, but now I had a safe place to fall again. I was coming to know a form of love that had the power to soothe and heal, even from the wounds I was suffering. I wondered what other surprises life had in store for me, but I wasn't afraid anymore.

When I thought back to the conditional nature of Dad's love, I no longer judged him. There is no denying the powerful impact of our relationship on my life, or how deeply I loved him. I know Dad loved me the best he could, and what he learned of love was based upon the models of love he had in his family. Most of the time, that was enough. I hope my children find peace in the fact that I, too, did my best. I hope these days they would say I'm doing better.

So I ask you now to reflect. Would you say you apply the principles of unconditional love to yourself? Do you accept yourself or are you critical? Can you come to terms with the hurtful and traumatic things that have happened over your lifetime so that you can love yourself now, as you are?

What was the most recent act of unconditional love you demonstrated to yourself or others? Are you or someone you love in need of a safe place to fall right now, and what can you do to fill that need in yourself or another?

You might want to pick up your journal and write. Or you might just want to pick up the phone and call someone you know who could benefit from a little unconditional love right about now.

CHAPTER 8

Trauma and the Loss of Safety

"If you want to improve the world, start by making people feel safer."

—STEPHEN PORGES

THE LOSS OF SAFETY IS ONE OF THE MOST SHOCKING CONSEQUENCES of trauma we suffer, whether from a single devastating incident or through gradual and repeated circumstances. Instead of feeling secure, we are overwhelmed with terrifying thoughts and feelings.

We may withdraw, be irritable, or become aggressive. The body may react as if the threat remains when it doesn't. We may avoid situations that remind us of the trauma. We do not feel safe even in circumstances that are safe, and with people who are there to protect and help us. Regaining a sense of safety is at the very center of our recovery from trauma. It is difficult to understand what happens to us psychologically or physiologically when we live in a world that no longer feels safe to us.

One of the cases Norm and I worked on together exemplifies what the loss of safety can look like in an abusive workplace setting. In this setting, employees had been suffering for years under a tyrannical boss, and many never felt safe. Even on weekends or time away from work, they felt the fear of their return to the office.

By the time we got involved, the damage already done was incalculable. The inability of a company executive to control her continuous angry, unpredictable, and bullying behaviors and the suffering of others became too much for one brave manager to bear, and he made a formal complaint to the board of directors.

If the complaints we were brought in to investigate by the company's general counsel were as pervasive and aggressive as they were described to be, they would constitute a widespread, corrosive, and hostile work environment where no one felt safe.

After a full week of interviews, Norm and I were alarmed by the high levels of stress and trauma the 25 people we spoke with were suffering. They had been robbed of any sense of well-being. Many had developed serious physical and psychological illnesses. They felt unsafe, and they were.

When we asked people what was triggering their fears, they said it was their love for their jobs, their concerns for coworkers, their boss's anger, and her power over their lives and livelihood. They were suffering to the point that we felt helpless. We came too late with too little we could do but listen and report. Maybe at least we could put an end to the reign of terror by their abuser.

Men and women sobbed as they spoke with us. They needed frequent breaks to compose themselves so they could continue. They were both scared and paranoid, looking around the room furtively for hidden microphones. They expressed fear regarding the impact of even talking to us and wondered what repercussions they would suffer despite our repeated assurances that no retaliation would be tolerated.

They panicked at the thought that they would be spotted coming or going from the meeting place we had designated. They parked their cars blocks away and walked to the interview location, came and went through side entrances, even disguising their appearances or pulling the hoods of their jackets up to hide their faces.

Dr. Stephen W. Porges, a distinguished scientist, authored the book *The Pocket Guide to the Polyvagal Theory: The Transformative Power of Feeling Safe.* The title of his work is off-putting, I know, but don't let it scare you. Dr. Porges explains how our neural circuitry supports our social behavior, interactions with others, and the ability for emotional regulation. Only when our nervous system judges that the environment we are in is safe can we begin to heal.

Safety is crucial to enabling us to be our best, optimize our potential, and live fulfilling and meaningful lives, argues Dr. Porges. Our reactions to the traumas we have experienced may fade over time, and we make positive adjustments in our lives. But when we are under stress again, we may experience that we are being retraumatized.

"Safe states are a prerequisite not only for social behavior but also for accessing the higher brain structures that enable humans to be creative and generative," Dr. Porges writes. Feeling safe again, regaining some sense of control and freedom from danger, is critical to the process of recovery and healing.

In order to find safety after it's lost, we have to understand what it is that disrupts our sense of safety, whether it is within ourselves, with others, or in the world around us. Living in a world that we, and our nervous systems, deem unsafe takes a great toll on us. We put up our defenses. We are afraid to be vulnerable. We shut down.

We may be drawn to stay in relationships that are not safe out of the fear of leaving. We may avoid getting into relationships that actually are safe because we fear intimacy or don't want to get hurt. The impact of trauma remains in control of many of our actions and keeps us from the comfort of a healthy mind and healthy relationships.

When we feel unsafe, it's hard to trust, it's hard to heal. We get anxious, paranoid, or depressed. It's hard to feel the benefits of unconditional love when we don't feel safe. The very connections we need with others remain elusive when we need them most.

As we understand our vulnerabilities to danger or the threatening of our lives, we have to start respecting the importance of intimate relationships. If we have lost trust in ourselves or others, we have to regain it. If we don't, we run the risk of dampening the defensive systems that allow us to form strong bonds with others.

Dr. Porges' words describe an enlightened understanding of safety and the deep trauma of losing it. He states, "Embedded in the social engagement system is our biological quest for safety and an implicit biological imperative to connect and co-regulate our physiologic state with another."

It is not just a loss we feel emotionally and psychologically; it is an actual loss of safety that is experienced in our body's nervous system as exemplified by the behaviors of those traumatized individuals I spoke of earlier in this chapter. We have, as Dr. Porges describes, a deep biological need to connect and calm or regulate our nervous system response with others who will enable the return to safety that is essential to our healing.

How we look at each other is a critical feature of this capacity to connect. Subtle cues of understanding, eye contact, active listening, shared feelings, and intentions are conveyed as we interact with others. Only when we are in a calm state physiologically can we actually express cues of safety to another.

It is our ability to create opportunities to genuinely connect and co-regulate with others that will determine the success of relationships after suffering trauma. So often we hear of couples who have lost a child, for instance, whose marriage cannot survive the tragedy. Rather than being drawn together, they have been torn apart. There is often a shutting down and a tendency toward isolation that occurs post-trauma when what we need to regain trust and a sense of safety comes from our interactions with others. When we don't feel safe, we are unable to make those around us feel safe.

The social engagement system provides us not only with the chance to express our own physiological state but also the opportunity to detect levels of distress or safety in others. Dr. Porges reminds us that, "When detecting safety, physiology calms. When detecting danger, physiology is activated for defense."

Safe states are critical to the establishment of well-being, social relatedness, and connection as we strive to overcome the negative consequences of trauma. Sometimes we assume we know what safety means, but it is important to examine the inconsistencies between the words we use to describe our bodily feelings of safety and what we are actually experiencing physiologically. We may be getting cues that we are ignoring or imaging things that are not true.

Sometimes we want to change, but we defend ourselves to avoid making ourselves vulnerable to being hurt or because we feel unsafe for some reason. For example, it was not easy to let Norm in at a time when I felt so unsafe, yet my interactions with him and his ability to connect, comfort, and accept me began to reverse the isolation I was experiencing at the time.

My interactions with him stirred me to trust again and told me: This is a safe place to fall. You can trust this person. I knew what it felt like to feel safe again. I knew what it felt like to be loved unconditionally. My nervous system calmed. It was undeniable. It was like coming home. It is a state of being essential to our deepest biological needs.

Below is a diagram of Dr. Porges' that depicts how he views the autonomic nervous system. I would suggest that you find a quiet place to reflect on this visual. Or you may want to take a few moments to close your eyes and bring to mind someone in your life who you feel safe with. How do you feel in their presence, and what about that person contributes to those feelings? Does your physiology calm and allow you to be vulnerable because you have the sensation of being safe?

Porges' View of the ANS
The Metaphor of Safety

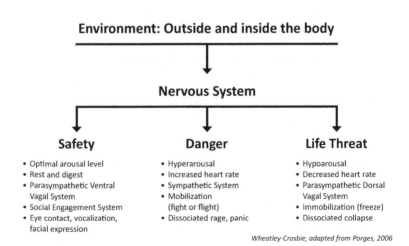

Environment: Outside and inside the body

↓

Nervous System

Safety	Danger	Life Threat
• Optimal arousal level	• Hyperarousal	• Hypoarousal
• Rest and digest	• Increased heart rate	• Decreased heart rate
• Parasympathetic Ventral Vagal System	• Sympathetic System	• Parasympathetic Dorsal Vagal System
• Social Engagement System	• Mobilization (fight or flight)	• Immobilization (freeze)
• Eye contact, vocalization, facial expression	• Dissociated rage, panic	• Dissociated collapse

Wheatley-Crosbie, adapted from Porges, 2006

As you can see, creating safety within and around us is critical to feeling safe again after suffering trauma or reinjury from the original trauma. We must relearn to trust ourselves in relationships with others if we seek to trust someone else. We have to learn to love ourselves unconditionally to feel safe and provide safety for others.

The process by which each of us regains a sense of safety is different, but the drive will keep pushing us forward until we find our way into the arms of safe people, places, and circumstances again. Real change comes from our ability to relax our defenses and co-regulate with others we trust. Those skills will also allow us to calm ourselves in moments of stillness and quiet reflection.

Reflecting now, what does safety mean to you? How do you calm yourself? How are you going to reclaim safety in your life?

PART III

From Trauma
to Transformation

CHAPTER 9

In the Aftermath of Trauma

"It is my intention to avoid the many perpetrator-victim dynamics
embedded in traumatized and traumatizing
societies all around me as much as possible,
and not foster any new perpetrator-victim dynamics myself."

—FRANZ RUPPERT

THE SUFFERING I EXPERIENCED WITH THE DEATH OF MY FATHER AND
the realization of the absence of connection and safety in my family
presented a challenging reality. Yet, over the years, my life has been
transformed in tremendously positive ways, as evidenced by my
healing, the discovery of unconditional love, and the trajectory of
my career. Who could have imagined it? Certainly not me!

If you look back to a traumatic experience or circumstance in your
life, when the future appeared bleak and your sense of loss or fear
overwhelmed you, what do you see? Do you recall a time when you
started to accept what had happened and you realized life would go
on? What were the things that helped you move on, and who were
the people who helped you feel safe again?

And do you remember a time when someone close to you suffered a
painful event or tragedy, and you provided them with a safe place to
fall? What cues were you able to give to them that you were safe and

could be trusted? There is no greater gift than knowing you helped someone else in their time of greatest need.

Big Trauma on a Big Stage

After working with Norm at Lifesource during the height of AIDS/ HIV, I needed a break from death and dying, or at least that's what I told myself. I started working for U.S. Behavioral Health in 1987. The company, now called United Behavioral Healthcare, provided employee assistance and managed mental health care programs to corporate clients and government agencies.

I was hired as the National Director of Training, Education, and Consultation. I built the department and the programs we delivered over my seven years with the company. My team had responsibilities that included nationwide critical incident response, employee and management training, sexual harassment prevention, and stress and conflict management. Little did I know that I would have another encounter with violence, or that this time it would be on an un-imaginable scale.

On Thursday, July 1, 1993, I was driving across the Golden Gate Bridge in the middle of the afternoon. All the windows were down; the air was salt-scented. I had left my office at U.S. Behavioral Health earlier than usual to jump-start the long and welcomed holiday weekend. On the radio, the Beatles blared "Good Day, Sunshine." The music and wind almost drowned out the ringing of my phone, but at the last minute, I answered.

It was my assistant, Donna. "Thank God you answered. I have

Susan on the phone from Pettit & Martin. There's an active shooter in their offices. I'll patch her through." With that, Donna was gone.

At the time, my team was working on a project for Pettit & Martin, a real estate law firm, located at 101 California Street, in the heart of San Francisco's financial district. Pettit & Martin's human resources manager, Susan, was now on the line as I pulled onto our carport and turned off the engine.

As she began to speak, I felt a stomach punch and instantly knew that this was a call that was going to change my life again, like the call I received from my mother all those years ago. Susan said, in a voice laced with hysteria that sometimes broke up her words, "Someone started shooting up the office. He's still here. He's running floor to floor and the bullets are—" and then she stopped midsentence as another bullet was fired. This one I heard, too.

Now I felt the hair on the back of my neck stand up and the pattern of my breathing change. The human resources professionals I'd come to know and respect in recent months, and the others who sought shelter with them, may be close to the end of their lives, I thought.

"Are you alright?" I asked as the shooting seemed to subside.

"Yes, but I don't know what's going on out there. We are barricaded in the personnel office and some of the staff is here with us. We pushed the file cabinets in front of the door. We're going to need you."

Then, on the line, I could hear loud knocking and then, "San Francisco Police. Is anyone in there?"

A rattling noise followed, and I heard multiple voices gasping. Susan drew a deep breath. She said, "Oh my god. The door opens outward. We were sitting ducks. Thank God it's the police and not the shooter." Hurriedly, she added, "I've got to go. I'll call you back as soon as I can. Please stand by," and the phone went dead.

My training, education, and experience provided the qualifications I needed to respond to this traumatic event of shocking proportions. But it was the senseless murder of my father that uniquely prepared me to assist in the aftermath of the shooting at 101 California Street.

In those early moments and the months that followed, I could see the straight line that marked my journey from November 20, 1976, to July 1, 1993. Though I was more prepared and better trained now, nothing could have prepared anyone for the violence that tore through the beautiful glass and concrete skyscraper with its 360-degree view of San Francisco Bay.

After Susan ended the call, I sat in the car for a few minutes wondering how many people would die that day at Pettit & Martin and how many more lay wounded. My mind racing, I gathered my purse and briefcase and headed into the house to await further information.

On TV, the images flashing on the screen were horrific; the words were even worse. At 2:57 p.m., Gian Luigi Ferri, a 55-year-old mortgage broker, had casually entered one of the high-rise elevators, carrying a gym bag. As he neared the 34th floor, Ferri unzipped his bag and laid out his weapons: two TEC-9 semi-automatic pistols and a Norinco NP44, a Chinese-manufactured copy of a Colt M1911 semi-automatic pistol.

The report said that Ferri also had hundreds of rounds of ammunition and a serious grudge against certain lawyers who worked at the firm. As the doors parted, he was said to have been startled by a firm secretary who had pressed the button for the elevator.

Ferri did not shoot the woman. Instead, he instructed her not to move. He had a target list of lawyers in his pocket that he believed failed him in a business transaction 12 years prior.

He was a killer on a mission. He had loaded weapons in his gym bag, which he carried as he walked down a short passageway.

He stopped in front of a glass-enclosed conference room where a deposition regarding a sex discrimination lawsuit was being held. There were five people in the room. Ferri killed two of them. He reportedly walked past the bank of secretaries and roamed the 34th floor, where he shot more victims before moving down an interior flight of stairs to the floor below.

By the time Susan called back, Ferri had murdered eight people and injured six others before he took his own life as the police closed in on him.

Untold others were traumatized by the actions of this deranged man seeking revenge for the failings of his own life. San Francisco was stunned that day. The shootings at Pettit & Martin were like the beginning of an epidemic. The workplaces where we once felt safe, no longer were. Schools and campuses across the country where we thought our children were safe, no longer were.

Until 1993, workplace violence, other than during the execution of a robbery or crime in high-risk businesses like banks or at post offices, was exceedingly rare. After 1993, it became a frequent occurrence. Although I had spent the last seven years dealing with a variety of complex human dramas in workplaces across the country, this was my first experience with the phenomenon.

Facing one of my professional life's most challenging and defining moments, I was able to rely on my training on the work of Jeffrey Mitchell and his Critical Incident Stress Debriefing (CISD) model. I knew even then that, somehow, Dad had a hand in my new career. His brutal death and my response to it were part of my hands-on training that would serve me in the days that were to follow.

Transforming Trauma

That evening I was able to mobilize the internal resources I needed to address the trauma of others. I had an amazing team of people to support me in efforts to confront this unspeakable drama that had just taken place. My intention was to create a zone of safety where vulnerabilities would be treated with compassion and caring.

Pettit & Martin administrators reserved the ballroom at the San Francisco Park Hyatt Hotel for a 9 a.m. debriefing session we were planning for the next morning. My gut and my training in the Mitchell model told me that waiting to respond to the tragedy until after the long holiday weekend was not an option.

Bringing those who had suffered this horrific event together as soon as possible was the only thing that made sense to me from a human and psychological perspective. Time is not on your side following such a Big Trauma. Everyone involved needed a safe place to fall, and fast.

Shock quickly sets in, fear grows, unanswered questions multiply, and faulty facts fill in for the truth. I knew all too well how important it was to address head-on the sense of survivor's guilt people would be feeling and the self-recrimination that comes when we start to second-guess our actions.

When people die or are wounded around you but your life is spared, wild thoughts race through your mind. You ask yourself, "Why not me?" You wonder what action you should have taken. It's not a good cycle to get into, and only seems to compound the tragedy you just lived through.

I wanted to do what I could to avoid that downward spiral for the survivors. Later that evening, a group voicemail was sent to the entire firm. We had no idea how many people would check their messages that evening or show up the following morning. We just knew that we would be there and that it was the right thing to do if we were to help the healing begin. Donna and I spent the rest of the evening fielding calls from Pettit & Martin leadership and U.S. Behavioral Health colleagues.

I thought of the lessons Norm had taught me about the power of unconditional love, especially in times of great sorrow. I imagined finding a way to replicate the comfort of his famous group hugs in the shared experience we were planning for the following day.

I knew that the emotions would grow in intensity as the reality of the horror settled in overnight. It is only the sociopath or the very disturbed among us that has a nonresponse to committing or responding to violent acts. For the rest of us, there is no neutral in the face of senseless murder.

In the aftermath of such acts, what emerges is either the best or the worst in each of us. We come together, as was occurring already at Pettit & Martin, or we turn on each other and escape into our own worlds. We took our first steps toward finding safety in the aftermath of extreme trauma and fear.

I am left to wonder how many among you—my readers—have been touched by these kinds of traumas, where you work, in the schools your children attend, or in the communities where you live. I wonder who was there for you and how your life was changed forever after. I wonder if you had a safe place to fall, as we hoped to provide for these survivors.

Coming Together to Heal

After a short, restless night, I was relieved when Friday morning dawned. I showered and readied myself for a solemn day. Donna picked me up and when we arrived at the hotel an hour early, the lower lobby was already filling with grief-stricken mourners. Some sat on couches while others stood together in small circles in corners. I watched as they held each other, cried together, and shared their stories in hushed tones—some afraid, I suspected, to hear their own words.

As I watched people gather, I had no idea what I was going to say. I found a place in a far corner to wait alone. I'm not embarrassed to tell you that I used the wall for support. I was afraid that without it, I would fall into a nearby chair and not find the courage to rise again and comfort the crowd.

From where I stood in this massive ballroom meant for celebrations filled with gaiety, I could see that the mood this morning would be somber and dark. I had a clear view of people as they filtered in until the room was overflowing. By the time we were to begin, there were over 250 attorneys, staff, and family members present.

I moved from the corner of the room to the center of the stage and surveyed the crowd as hundreds of eyes searched mine, looking for answers and awaiting a comforting voice I wasn't sure I could find. I imagined Dad out there somewhere looking back at me. As I stood center stage, not certain how to cut through the dense fog of emotion in the room, unbidden thoughts of my father's murder and the morning after crowded my mind and refused to leave. Soft, silent tears rolled down my cheeks until I tasted the salt on the corners of my mouth. I could feel my father's presence in that room, and for a moment I found myself engulfed in his arms. And then I found the words.

"There is nothing I can say to you as a trained professional this morning that will do much good. But as the daughter of a murdered father and a mother who witnessed his murder and survived, I can be here with you, having been where you are."

And be there we were, for three intensely human and healing hours. There was no shortage of weeping or words. Unconditional love was flowing forth. I saw and felt the power of it that day in a way that opened my heart further as it calmed my mind.

We even found the courage to laugh at times and break up the heavy emotions into bearable chunks. The sheer volume of devastation, pain, and anger, and the cold chill of violence that hung in the room, left me breathless at times. But also in that room were vast amounts of humility, compassion, and love.

The flood of feelings released the pressure everyone had been under like a dam opening to let loose water that had risen to dangerous levels. The veil of denial we wear at times like this to mask the ugly face of violence was ripped away, and we confronted the truth together. We felt safe in our connectedness, in the telling of our stories, and the opportunity to help others.

We listened as people spoke of their personal experiences that day, sharing what they were doing when the shooting started, where they were, and what they witnessed. We talked about the friends they lost and the conditions of those who were injured. A mosaic of the massacre took shape as each piece of the puzzle was placed in a frame in our minds.

People wanted to know how this could have happened and what would happen next. They cheered colleagues who had acted heroically and saved the lives of others. They wanted to know, in the end, what they could do to help and who would be there to help them in the days ahead. In our shared vulnerabilities, we gained strength.

Together, we created an island of safety where they could break down and reach out in a world that had suddenly turned dangerous. I marveled at the miraculous strength, courage, and resilience displayed in that ballroom just hours after their lives had changed forever.

It was also undeniable for me to see that my life, for the second time, had been dramatically altered by sudden, unforeseeable events. I knew that I was on a new path that I could never have predicted. When the meeting ended, one of the attendees pulled me aside and said, "When we heard about your father, we knew we were in good hands."

I am hopeful that within the traumas we each suffer there also exists the opportunity to change in ways that bring value to others even as we heal. Whether you pull out your journal, go for a walk in nature, call a friend, or meditate, take a few minutes to reflect on where you are in your life and how far you've come. If you look deeply within, can you identify for yourself the ways in which your trauma has led to opportunities to make the world a better and safer place for others?

I have learned over and over again throughout the years just how precious life is. I have also had the experience of life changing without warning. There is no time like the present to appreciate where you are and what and who in your surroundings give you solace and feelings of safety.

CHAPTER 10

Facing Down Fear

"Fear makes come true that which one is afraid of."

—Victor E. Frankl

Our fears can keep us stuck in trauma longer than they need to. When we fight or deny our fears, they maintain their power over us and slow the path to recovery. The reality is that there is no way to move through fear other than to feel it. After all, it is the nature of feelings to be felt. That is their reason for being.

When we are in the midst of trauma, our psyche protects us from feeling the depth of our fears. They would only serve to immobilize us. When, however, we are ready to move toward healing, that movement can carry us beyond the dark territories trauma took us to and lead us onto the road to feeling safe again.

I've learned to trust the natural and rhythmic patterns of healing that take place in the human mind if we remain open and present in every moment. I've experienced them in myself, and I've witnessed those patterns countless times in others who I have worked with over the years.

One particular story of survival at Pettit & Martin touched me deeply. Most of us go to great lengths in our lives to avoid our deepest fears and darkest memories. And yet, when we least expect it, what frightens us most finds us, and we are forced to face it.

Lew's Story

Lew had no way to prepare for the danger he would face on the 33rd floor of Pettit & Martin. He cheated death that day and lived to share his story. We spent many long hours working together in the months that followed the shootings.

Unfortunately, over the years, Lew and I lost touch with each other, as too often happens in my work. I connect deeply with unbelievably brave and courageous people in the midst of their most harrowing moments, and then they fade away and we disappear from each other's lives.

While writing this book, I sought to locate Lew in 2019. I wanted his permission to share his story. More than anything, I wanted to know how he was doing. I knew from my trauma work and personal life that what Lew went through was life-altering. It would not only influence the rest of his life but would always be with him like it happened yesterday. When I reached him by phone, our voices were overcome with emotion. It was as if the last 25 years had not passed at all.

The gratitude that flowed from him touched me deeply. The fact that he was happily married and living in a remote, peaceful place made me smile. On the other side of fear, Lew found unconditional love that helped him heal. He found a safe place to fall. I hoped to learn how he was able to do that.

Lew now had a mediation practice in a small town, helping the people in his community find peaceful resolution to differences. There were no high-rise buildings, no crazed, angry clients. Lew gave me permission to share his story, and we made plans to see each other when he would be visiting in the Bay Area.

But for now, allow me to introduce you to the Lew I first met. On July 1, 1993, he had been working on a contracted basis for several months at Pettit & Martin, where he sat in a small office on the mostly empty 33rd floor. He was in the process of securing a permanent position as a mediator for the U.S. Court of Appeals.

Lew and I met at his Richmond, California, home while he was recovering from his injuries. Lew started our interview by saying, "It was a weird day. My morning was routine. I was reviewing documents at my desk. I had a late lunch with a woman I was dating. We had a little fight while we were eating. When we walked back to 101 and were standing by the revolving doors to the building, I gave her a little lecture about the importance of not living your life with too much regret. It was eerie," Lew said. "I remember telling her that life is too short and that we never know how long we are going to live. I told her that there wasn't enough time for us to waste worrying about bad haircuts. And then, within moments of that conversation, I was faced with the pivotal issue as to whether I would live or I would die."

Upstairs, working at his desk, Lew suddenly heard shooting outside his office door and an armed man appeared in the doorway.

"I thought to myself that this is not the time for me to die. I had too many things I hadn't done yet that I wanted to do," Lew said. "I wasn't willing to die that day. I wasn't ready to die. Those are the thoughts that were going through my mind in a split second."

Lew was quiet for a moment before continuing. He said, "I was sitting there behind the desk and this guy just started shooting me ... Whatever I had to do I was going to do. I wasn't going to die."

Lew continued with his story. "I don't remember how I got out of the room. I just did."

"I ducked into another office. I called 911 and had a brief, one-way conversation. Then I hung up and called this woman Allison. I told her to cancel the barbeque I was supposed to have that night at my house. Then I was quiet for 20 minutes or so. I felt that whatever was happening on this floor was over."

When Lew saw police officers and firefighters coming out of the freight elevator, he knew he would be okay and that he had survived his worst fears that day. He was whisked into the elevator and down to the lobby. People were laid out near him; emergency people were working on them. "I fell into shock then," Lew said. "I stopped working on being in control. I finally felt safe."

The next thing Lew remembered was being wheeled toward an ambulance. "I was in the intake cubicle talking to a nurse when a Dominican nun walked in to console me. She wanted to contact my family, but I didn't want her to. I just thought that I would do it myself when I got home." But Lew wasn't released that day. He had one surgery that afternoon and another the following day.

He said, "I remember a firm partner who came by to see how I was. I had a horde of visitors over the next day or two. It was like being at my own wake. It was like people hardly ever are in real life, telling me how much they appreciate me, how much they loved me. I must have had 20 to 30 people visit me in two or three days before I was released to go home."

Reunion and Recovery

Lew and I had our reunion at a coffee shop near my home in Marin County. I found him sitting under the shade of a wonderful old oak, sipping his coffee. I couldn't hold back my smile and neither could Lew. He stood up and we hugged each other. As we sat down, soft tears began to fall; both of us were touched by the presence and survival of the other.

Lew had made many changes and decisions in the years since the events at Pettit & Martin that marked his path to safety and healing. He recovered from his injuries, taking the time he needed to do so. When he did return to work, it was in a different environment in an area of the law that was less litigious and competitive.

He was able to build a strong support system, confront old areas of dysfunction, and find an unconditionally loving woman who accepted him as he was, with all his wounded parts. They were married and moved to a quieter place, living a life that they had chosen, free from the dangerous streets of San Francisco.

Lew was grateful for his new life. He and his wife took the time to travel around the world, a dream he always had. He didn't hide from his fears when they resurfaced, and he was able to balance the trauma with love, self-understanding, and time in nature. Lew had found a safe environment and a renewed appreciation for the gift of life.

I can tell you that from my perspective, Lew made changes and decisions, created a lifestyle, and joined a community wherein he feels safe. He was, however, changed forever, and when you think about it, how could one not be? Why would a person want to remain unchanged after such a close call with death?

We can't erase the violence, but we can recover, move forward, and live meaningful lives. We can seek out safe places to fall and find them. We can learn to trust and welcome unconditional love into our hearts. We can live the dreams we once abandoned.

My work with the Pettit & Martin team—and with Lew, in particular—was deeply gratifying and healing. To this day, hanging in my office is the framed memento they presented to me. It is titled "With deep appreciation from Pettit & Martin." It has the signatures of and messages from many of the people who I worked with during that year.

When you look back on your life, would you say you fear or welcome change, even when it's unexpected or caused by traumatic events? When a new opportunity comes your way, do you seize it or turn away from it? Remember, you have the power to choose what you do next at this moment, with this day, with those you love, and in the years ahead. By way of a little inspiration and motivation, I share with you the well-tested wisdom of Dr. Assagioli and his focus in Psychosynthesis on free will.

When asked in an interview to describe the will, Assagioli responded, "At some point, perhaps in a crisis when danger threatens, an awakening occurs in which the individual discovers his will. This revelation that the self and the will are intimately connected can change a person's whole awareness of himself and the world. He sees that he is a living subject, an actor, endowed with the power to choose, to relate, and to bring changes in his own personality."

Take a moment to think about what Assagioli is saying above. How does your experience of trauma and recovery relate to the power of free will? Were you able to make choices and changes that led you from trauma to opportunity?

Trauma and Opportunity

After the mass shooting at Pettit & Martin and the recovery efforts that followed, on September 1, 1993, I tendered my resignation to U.S. Behavioral Health and started a career as an independent consultant, continuing my work with the Pettit & Martin team.

I was interviewed on radio and television, wrote and published articles, and was asked to speak to large groups and universities. In the course of a few months, I gained a national reputation as one of the foremost experts on workplace violence at a time and in a field where there weren't many of us and the need was exploding.

When I was asked to make a presentation in Washington, D.C. to a group of union and business leaders about workplace violence and mental health, I invited Mom to come with me. We had a lot of healing to do. We were at our best together when it was just the two of us. That was when our compatibility and caring were not restricted or distorted by our family's dysfunction. We stopped first in New York and were able to speak more frankly about her trauma and loss, and my own.

I shared my experiences with her about the brave people I met at Pettit & Martin, and Mom shared her story of survival with me. My heart opened toward my mother on that trip, and I saw a strength in her I hadn't seen when Dad was alive. She was not only surviving now, she was thriving.

It seemed that during her years with her second husband, Bill, Mom had come into her own and moved out of the shadow of Dad's death. Their relationship, I had to admit, made Mom happier than I remembered her being with Dad.

Bill had a wonderful sense of humor that Dad did not have. They traveled the world together and had adventures that made her life richer and perhaps, somehow, eased some of the suffering she had experienced.

In D.C., as I made my presentation, I looked out at the audience and saw the pride on my mother's face. I had waited a very long time to experience that moment. After the presentation, she said, "Bobbi, I'm so proud of you and who you've become."

One tragedy had created an opportunity for the healing of another. The perfect merging of two seemingly unrelated violent events spanned 17 years of my life. In some strange way, Dad's death gave me purpose as I moved on with my life and into a career that I seemed destined to follow.

Amid all the change, in November 1993, my life was blessed by the birth of my first grandchild, the daughter of my daughter. I was gratefully reminded of the full cycle of life, from birth to death, which remains unchanged in the shadow of tragedy.

Then, in January 1994, Norm approached me with a new proposal. We were ready for a new challenge and the opportunity to work together again. We were inspired to form our own corporation, Confidante, Inc. and set out to not only prevent workplace violence and other traumatic events but to also become "creators of workplace harmony." Beginnings and endings followed one another closely. My life, it seemed, was in continuous motion.

CHAPTER 11

The Path to Healing

"In the last analysis, the individual person is responsible for
living his own life and for 'finding himself.'
If he persists in shifting his responsibility to somebody else,
he fails to find the meaning of his own existence."

—THOMAS MERTON

IF WE ARE TO TRULY HEAL FROM THE TRAUMAS WE HAVE SUFFERED, IT is critical that we understand the cycles of reinjury that all too often victimize or imprison us. If we don't look at the roots of our trauma, we can't break the cycle. We continue to reinjure ourselves and those we love. An essential part of the healing journey involves self-reflection and the uncovering of truths once buried but not forgotten. You hold the keys to unlocking the mysteries of yourself and gaining freedom from the past.

The psychological impact of the traumas each of us has experienced over our lifetimes creates "black holes" in our personal biographies that are maintained in our unconscious and drive our behaviors in unseen ways. If you review your own childhood, can you identify a time when you felt victimized by someone? With the passage of time, did you find yourself in a position of power over that person or someone else, and feel yourself step into the shoes of the perpetrator?

The Victim-Perpetrator Cycle

Dr. Ruppert has done a great deal of groundbreaking work related to the victim-perpetrator cycle. He also has developed a treatment methodology called Identity-Oriented Psychotrauma Therapy. This therapy allows us to reconnect with our experiences of victimhood so that we can recognize our victim attitudes and how they impact our lives.

Working with a therapist trained in Ruppert's theories and studying on my own, I realized that my deepest fears and childhood victim persona were very much alive. Yet I did not consciously identify my adult self as a victim or a perpetrator or fully grasp the ways in which I continued to reinjure myself and breathe new life into old traumas.

For the most part, I had successfully established healthy relationships and a rewarding, successful career. And yet I was reminded that the toxic, negative relationships of the past, such as those between abusers and their abused partners, cast a dark shadow on the present that is difficult to escape.

While writing this book over the last few years and continuing to explore past traumas, I ran into parts of myself that hadn't participated in my healing, until now. It was stunning to realize that while I had faced the Big Trauma of Dad's death and helped the traumatized victims at Pettit & Martin, I hadn't successfully faced the wounded child in me or the family dysfunction that I had somehow normalized.

I assure you, there are some unpleasant surprises in store for you as you take your own journey, but it's best that you don't avoid them or wait for another trauma to shake you to your core. I also assure you, there is no way out of long-buried feelings of pain and anger other than straight through them.

Dr. Ruppert's recent book, *Who Am I in a Traumatised and Traumatising Society*, helped me restore, recover, and repair the child of dysfunction and conditional love alive in me. I learned from his work that if any of us truly wants to lead a life beyond the perpetrator-victim dynamics, we can only do so if we remove ourselves from the relationship system in which we have become trapped.

I want to share with you a powerful quote from Dr. Ruppert on the subject. He says, "A child cannot yet leave a loveless family, and the withdrawal from a traumatising partnership is most often not possible in one day. However, anyone who has recognized the perpetrator-victim cycle in which he or she is caught will at least be motivated to exit it, and will use every possible opportunity to do so."

I was motivated indeed, but I had to face hard truths I had long avoided that were still alive and buried memories of early trauma and family drama. Are you caught in the perpetrator-victim cycle somewhere in your life and are you motivated to remove yourself from it? Are you currently part of an unhealthy family dynamic that you know isn't healthy for you? Awareness of these dynamics as they relate to your own experience is the first crucial step to change. You simply can't change what you don't accept needs to be different.

Breaking the Cycle

Breaking the cycle involves taking responsibility for our own behavior and recognizing the roles we play in cycles of dysfunction.

I know that I am the only one who can break the victim-perpetrator cycle for me as you are for yourself. Each one of us who does so makes it that much easier for the next person to break free. Think about it this way: There will be one less person contributing to the trauma in your life and to our traumatized society, and one healthier person to partner up with.

It's important that we focus on developing our own healthy self and pay attention to our own needs. We need to—for our own good—exit the recurring and unhealthy victim-perpetrator cycle Dr. Ruppert describes. We so often recreate the very traumas we desperately want to escape. Instead, we need to create healthy autonomy and clear boundaries for ourselves.

We may exit a relationship to escape victimization only to repeat the cycle elsewhere in our lives. We carry with us the attitudes of victimhood that we internalized as a result of traumatic episodes we suffered at the hands of perpetrators over our lifetimes.

Herein lies one of the great gifts of self-reflection and inner healing. We get to the root of our faulty thinking so that we can free ourselves from it. We learn to resist the pull of the victim mentality that was once an acquired personality trait that led us into damaging interactions or relationships. For example, I thought I was free of my sister when I exited the relationship, but I wasn't. It was the victim in me from which I needed freedom. It was exiting the cycle itself that broke the chain of dysfunction. Unfortunately, it wasn't until my mother died at age 102 that I was finally able to make a clean break from Ann and, eventually, from the cycle itself.

I have often wondered why I waited, what took me so long to break the cycle of dysfunction I had been trapped in most of my life.

I hope you don't wait as long as I did to shine the light into yourself and set the victimized child in you free.

Trapped in the Past

One childhood memory haunted me as I grieved for my mother and sought to understand myself better. We had a cat when I was six years old. For the life of me, I cannot remember his name or whether we had him long enough to give him one. The trauma, however, I do remember.

As I mentioned earlier, growing up I had a small room in the farthest corner of the second floor of the big house on 18th Avenue. My sister had the entire third floor, with a regulated stairway I couldn't climb without permission. You could say I looked up to her or she looked down on me—literally.

I loved the third floor, especially the playroom filled with toys, games, and a record player, but I didn't have the authority to go up there whenever I wanted to. I needed Ann's permission to go upstairs, and her invitations were rare.

One day, my brother found an abandoned kitten on his way home from school. He begged Mom to let him keep it. She did on one condition: The kitten, she insisted, had to live in the third-floor playroom and could not come out.

It was the job of my brother and sister to feed, clean, and play with the cat. It was fun for a while until my siblings lost interest. Then, I became the only one that cuddled and played with him, but that was only when I was given permission.

I would hear the cat crying and scratching at the door but I dared not go upstairs until my sister and brother got home from school. Even then, they would expel me after a short time when they went downstairs, and they never let me take him to my room.

However, sometimes, I did sneak up by myself when nobody was around. I even thought about setting the cat free. One day, I was home sick from school. When I went into the hallway outside my room, I heard terrible noises and what sounded like the cat bouncing off the door and walls. And then it became very still.

I made my way slowly up the stairs. When I opened the door, I found him dead on the other side of the room. I think he had literally gone crazy from loneliness and being caged up.

All the arbitrary rules killed the cat. You can keep the cat but only under these conditions. You can play with the cat but only when I say so. We want the cat but we don't want to take any responsibility for him. Like the love most frequently experienced in my family, it had conditions.

Losing my time with the kitty and considering the way he died was traumatic for me. I think, looking back, it was a lesson learned about conditional love and power. Somehow, in my mind, I knew I didn't have any. I don't know what the equivalent of the cat would be in human terms in my family, but I sure didn't want to find out.

I imagine in some families being the youngest child is a cherished position to hold. That wasn't my experience. Perhaps my early childhood experiences prepared me to face bullies and aggressors in the workplace. I've defended innocent victims and confronted their perpetrators, but I could never face or free myself from my past or the pain suffered by the thoughtless acts of my family. I was definitely in the victim role, holding victim attitudes.

The bitterness I experienced, the anger that welled up in me as I reflected and wrote this segment, shocked me. Long-buried emotions revisited and overwhelmed me. I wondered how this could be with all the psychological and healing work I've done. How could I be so stuck, hurt, and angry? The psychological wounds still hadn't fully healed—proof that the impact of some traumas can last for a lifetime.

I was stuck in the vicious cycle of reinjury. I wanted to make my sister the victim. Maybe I was tired of being hurt and wanted to be the one to strike out for a change. I moved between roles but not out of the cycle. I hadn't exited the dynamics. I just changed places. I experienced the codependency that can develop between the victim and perpetrator roles. One needs the other to keep the cycle going.

I wanted to be the aggressor for a change. I was tired of being made to feel small. I wanted to be the self-righteous one. But that was merely a fantasy playing out in my mind, not something I ever acted upon.

By exposing the victim-perpetrator attitudes in my own psyche, my preoccupation with Ann gradually began to disappear. What happens as we bring these attitudes to our awareness is that we begin to free ourselves from the perpetrators in our lives. We no longer need to be understood, accepted, recognized, or loved by them.

We no longer need to exact justice from them, take revenge upon them, or enjoy the satisfaction of witnessing their misery. In the end, we don't need to stay stuck in our own victim attitudes that keep us engaged in a kind of dysfunctional dance with our wrongdoers.

When it comes to childhood trauma, nobody can make it different or better than it was, but we can come to accept it. I can't change how my mother loved me. I can't erase the way my sister treated me. You can't ignore the injustices done to you, nor can you make them okay or take the blame.

We can't turn judgment into acceptance, but that doesn't make it any less important that we come to terms with the past exactly as it was. While it is important to look back on those times of our lives, we are best served if we do that deliberately.

It's important to your own healing that you take the time you need for self-reflection. I invite you to sit quietly and imagine yourself stepping into your past and a time in childhood when you felt judged or scolded or unloved. How did you explain that experience to yourself then? Visualize yourself wrapping your inner child in a soft, warm blanket of unconditional love and acceptance now.

The Final Straw

What exactly happened to push me over the edge and bring an end to my victimization and, therefore, the need for a perpetrator to keep me in the cycle? The final straw came the day I went to say goodbye to my mother in her last hours of life and encountered Ann.

My eyes were wide open that day and I would have expected no less from my sister. I didn't fall into some magical thinking that this would be a moment of healing and coming together with Ann. I was not anyone's victim that day. Instead, I was a loving daughter there to say goodbye to my mother. My sister was the sideshow.

Ann was already sitting by Mom's bedside. I said hello, but she didn't respond. I sat across from her, on the other side of the bed. When I looked at her, the coldness in her eyes sent a chill through me as it often did when I was young.

I wondered what trauma she had suffered before I was born that made her into such an angry person. I wondered why her anger was directed at me and was never satiated, but I didn't feel victimized either.

I turned my attention to Mom. She wasn't moving. She laid there unconscious and far from the tension in the room, only hours from death. As far as I could tell, the part of her that mattered most was already gone. Her body didn't know I was there or what was happening around her.

Just then, my sister did a strange thing. She stretched her arms out and held her dog close to my mother. The dog licked Mom's closed eyes and colorless cheek. Then my sister looked my way. I knew that sitting in silence with me in the room was not really in her nature. I imagined her emotions must have felt like a toxic soup that threatened to boil over at any moment.

I didn't feel safe sitting across from her. But I was very grateful to be me and to feel the peace I felt with Mom. At that moment, I didn't envy Ann's closeness with Mom. Instead, I wondered if she would ever find peace or come to terms with the demons that drove her or if she ever really had the ability to care at all.

As I sat there lost in thought and stroking Mom's arm, Ann said out of the blue, "What kind of person are you?"

I asked, "What do you mean?"

She responded, that familiar shrillness in her voice, "I asked you what kind of person are you? There is something wrong with people like you who don't have a dog. If you don't have a dog to love nobody will ever love you. You're pathetic."

I didn't answer. I found comfort in memories of times when I sat with other siblings hovering over dying parents in the course of my work. I could recall their laughter, their tears, the comfort and warmth they gave to each other so naturally. I can honestly say that I had never heard a conversation of this nature at a deathbed vigil.

Just then, my son entered the room. He loved his grandmother completely and was one of her favorites. He stood at the foot of Mom's bed. His resemblance to Dad was unmistakable. He is six foot three and fit like Eddie. His face mirrored his grandfather's soft smile and gentle, loving eyes. I wondered if Mom could sense him there and feel Dad's energy.

My son stood there, holding on to the handrails of the hospital bed, fighting back tears. Silence had never been one of my sister's strengths. Ann turned to my son and said, "You know, your grandmother was the only real mother you ever had." She then pointed in my direction and said, "She wasn't a real mother to you. She's never been a mother to you. She doesn't love you."

My son and I said our goodbyes to Mom and left. There was comfort in our compassion for one another and the long hug we shared before getting into our cars and driving away.

I never saw Ann again after Mom's funeral. When her attacks continued as the trustee of my mother's estate, I hired an attorney. In the end, that was the resolution to our troubled relationship and the dissolution of my victim mentality. The child in me was healing. Unconditional love had replaced the conditional love I grew up with. I had safe places to fall.

Healing Ourselves

When I first assumed that my mother must love me because I was her child, I honestly thought that love was a birthright. After all, my father loved me from the beginning—why not my mother? Why did she demonstrate love and affection toward my siblings but ignore me and leave me to fend for myself?

I believed that being loved would naturally be afforded to me by, first and foremost, my mother who gave birth to me, followed closely by my father and siblings. It didn't turn out that way. I often wondered how I ended up in this family at all.

I don't believe anymore that a child is born into a family and, therefore, they are loved. I don't believe love is a birthright. Maybe that was one of the first lies I told myself when I was old enough to question or attempt to understand just what my family felt about me and me about them.

What exactly are we born into emotionally? Some children—the truly fortunate ones, like Norm—are born to unconditionally loving parents who have a healthy love to give that they inherited from past generations in their ancestry lines.

Maybe you had a healthy, beautiful foundation of unconditional love from day one of your life. If so, it was not because it was your birthright. Rather, it was because your parents were capable of giving those priceless gifts to you. And there is a high probability that they were raised with unconditional love in their lives.

With unconditional love, there is no blame, shame, or guilt. How different my life—any child's life—would be growing up surrounded by that kind of love. That doesn't mean we won't have our share of trauma in life or that we won't suffer pain and loss or tragedy. But it does mean that we will have the safety of unconditional love around us to catch us when we fall. We will also have the capacity to unconditionally love ourselves and others.

The majority of us were not born into welcoming arms and unencumbered love. Instead, we accept the conditional love that was given to us as our due. We embrace the flaws of our parents as our own shortcomings. We mold ourselves into the children we think they can love.

The trauma to self takes place in these early experiences, and during these years the cycle Ruppert describes begins. I found it easier to accept that I was undeserving than to see the source of the only love I knew as being flawed in some way. I had an investment in believing that how Dad loved me was perfect until I learned that it came with conditions.

It seemed to me that having Dad's love meant sacrificing the love of Mom and Ann and to a lesser extent, my brother. And Dad's love came at a high price. When I was 12, he would take me with him as cover when he went to meet his current girlfriend. I remember being the third wheel at lunch at the Fairmont Hotel, wondering what I was doing there.

I didn't feel special as I'd sit in the lobby reading a book while they disappeared and he later reappeared alone. It never seemed right to me but that was my role in his world. I easily took on the mantle of victimization. That is what it meant to be Daddy's "special girl" in my family.

And yet the expectancy I had of love is as natural as the sun rising every morning. We cry when we are babies out of a primal need to be held and loved. The response we receive is one of the primary markers for conditional or unconditional love.

What are your earliest recollections of being loved? Looking back, was it conditional or unconditional? Did it meet your expectations or fall short in some significant way?

These are critical questions because what we experience we call love. That's our model. It's how we love our life partners. That's how we love our children. The challenges we faced are the same challenges we create for those we love, even when those struggles are the opposite of what we want to create for them.

Thanks to Norm, I learned it doesn't have to be that way for your whole life. But it has been hard to break the cycle. It took years to realize that Ann's ability to love was flawed and damaged before I even came into the picture. Her feelings are likely reflections of her early traumas, which I will never know or understand. Finally, I realized that I didn't need to be victimized to find love where it doesn't exist. Neither do I need to strike out and hurt anyone else and become a perpetrator. These days, I am not as easily manipulated or corrupted by the need to be loved at all costs. It is the quality of love in our lives that heals and fortifies us, not the quantity of conditional love that we may have.

It's been freeing. Norm saw openness in me decades ago and a longing for true love long before I even knew it existed or was missing. My relationships with my children have changed for the better; my grandchildren are the epitome of the joys of giving and receiving unconditional love.

The gifts that Norm has given to me keep on giving. I remember how astounded he was by how I was treated by Mom and Ann. Norm worked hard over the years to teach me about the unqualified love I had always assumed was my birthright. What I understood about love in those early days of our relationship had nothing to do with the truth of love.

It wasn't until I learned through our experiences together that no matter what I did or how I hurt Norm or myself, his love for me was unwavering—his faith in me and his trust in me was unshakeable. I can't begin to count the number of times he has said to me over the years, "Don't be so mean to Bobbi."

Finally, ever so slowly, I have changed how I feel about myself, holding a healthier view of who I am and relating to those I am close to from a healthier, unconditionally loving and accepting place.

Can you love yourself in ways that you wanted others to and feel fulfilled? I hope so, and I know it's possible. It won't happen in one sitting, or you may already be there. Whatever the case, make a few notes in that journal and celebrate yourself. It's worth the time and tears. Unconditional love is foundational to the safe places and people you find on the path to healing.

As Dr. Ruppert advises, "Realize that there can be no higher authority than you in your life telling you what is good and right for you. You do not have to ask anyone for permission to live your own life.

It is your own life and only you can live it. Only you can find out what it means to live a good life for you."

I hope you find sanctuary in a safe place far from the perpetrator-victim cycle that trauma set in motion. I encourage you to take an honest look within your own psychological biography and shed new light and unconditional love on painful memories trapped within.

Take the words of Dr. Ruppert to heart. Take my experiences and words to heart. You don't have to ask permission of anyone to take these next steps on your own journey and open the door to the best years of your life.

PART IV

Obstacles to Healing

CHAPTER 12

Fate and Trauma

"When we look at our parents, then we see that behind them
are their parents, and behind their parents are other parents,
and so on through many generations. The same life flows
through all of them until it reaches us."

—Bert Hellinger

It is critical to confront the traumas that we have faced over our lives. It takes, however, a deeper dive into the generations that came before us to break free from the cycles of dysfunction and reinjury as we have discussed in prior chapters.

It is our inherited traumas often beyond our consciousness that drive us to repeat the fate of our ancestors. Gratefully, as we come to understand how we are impacted by generations past, we will be able to map out our path to personal freedom from their negative impact.

How many of you, I wonder, are aware of the pull of past generations on you now. We can fight fate, deny the power of it, or bow to it. Let me explain what I mean.

Dance with Fate

Fate, I realized, is what had already occurred in past generations of my family. I couldn't change the facts and events that have happened to me and before me, no matter how much I would like to do so. I knew I had to bow to and honor my fate and the sheer magnitude of its influence on my life. I was at a crossroads. I needed to accept what had already happened without judgment and learn from it without prejudice so that I could continue to carve a different future for myself and those I love.

After my mother died in 2014, I was introduced to Family Constellation Theory, which focuses on inherited family trauma and was developed by German psychotherapist Bert Hellinger. It is a way to discover the impact of underlying family bonds that carry over from past generations, unconsciously impacting us in the present.

It's a type of therapy that allows us to break generational patterns that unduly influence our lives. Family constellation can provide a new context of understanding ourselves and expand our understanding of human behavior and trauma in general.

According to Dr. Hellinger, bowing to fate can facilitate healing and is a way to honor that from which we came, which includes our parents and all of our ancestors. Fate, in constellation work, is understood as the larger context in which our individual and family lives unfold. Fate includes both good and bad fortune.

For example, I had the good fortune to have Dad's love. I had the misfortune to be robbed of it. My ancestors had the bad fortune to face the Holocaust and the violent loss of loved ones. I had the good fortune to be born in a different time. Just as I received gifts from fate, I also received hardships and challenges.

I learned that I could fight and reject my fate just as I could resist how and through whom life came to me. The negative feelings that were passed down to generations of women in my family range from entitlement, anger, jealousy, and competitiveness to resentment and rejection. Rather than changing fate, our feelings seemed to solidify the negative elements of our inheritance. They have been such a challenge to overcome.

I fought hard to have relationships that differed from those modeled in my family. My human connections weren't all that I wanted them to be or all that I knew they could be. I came to accept that no matter the form of the resistance I tested out at any given time, ultimately, I only weakened and isolated myself and strengthened the pull of fate that was dictating my future and changing nothing.

That's why Hellinger suggests an attitude of humility in the face of fate, hence the term "bowing" to it. That allows receptivity toward that which life has to give—a surrender to that which is. Only then, I realized, would I be able to accept the gift of life itself with all its many challenges and opportunities.

I ask you to think about inherited trauma in your own family. What patterns have repeated themselves over generations? What would it mean to you to bow to fate? What elements from your family history have had the greatest impact on your generation? What would it mean to you to surrender to fate?

For me, there was healing in surrender. I didn't feel so alone anymore. Fate, I believed, had my back. Receiving the truth of my fate as it wanted to flow through me, in exactly the way it was coming, brought with it the gift of unconditional love for self and others.

I thought of my ancestors and the impact of their lives on mine. They were stunning reminders of what we all struggle with: inherited emotional patterns and traumas that reach out to us through the mists of time and, sometimes, never let go. I realized that I didn't need to know exactly what happened in the past to my female ancestors to know that they had a profound impact on me in present time.

While they couldn't change their own fates or mine, I believed that I could move beyond them. I could lay down their burdens, which had become my own. I didn't need to die of the same affliction as my grandmother to honor her life. I didn't need to live out the dysfunction with my daughter that had been ingrained in us. I could be a model for and encourage my granddaughters to be instruments of change for the women of the future in my family.

I felt sadness for my grandmother, aunt, mother, and sister, for myself and my daughter and granddaughters. What was new was the empathy and compassion that arose in me. I thought about each of us hopelessly caught in this lonely and heartbreaking cycle, impervious to the unconditional love that surrounded us and that we were capable of giving to each other.

I felt the burden of present and past generations of women in my family firsthand. I prayed that somehow lightening my own would facilitate them to do the same for themselves. The possibilities for positive change seemed boundless but lay somewhere beyond me still.

Inherited Trauma

We've talked about Big Traumas and little traumas, pandemics, and other ongoing repetitive traumas. My discoveries about inherited trauma both complicated and clarified my prior understanding. I saw and experienced the dysfunctional patterns in my family, particularly among the women.

When I started this journey, I was not aware many of my struggles had their roots in another time. I don't think I fully grasped that fate was filled with potholes of trauma I was destined to fall into through no fault of my own. In my own studies and training in Family Constellation Theory and individual and group sessions with practitioners, I have come face to face with some harsh truths that have contributed in the end to my healing. I was reminded of every bit of the psychopathy I inherited.

In many respects, it is freeing to know that the roots of dysfunction started before you were even born. Bringing awareness to their current day influence on you may allow you to create a future that is different and healthier than predestined, unconscious drivers from the past. Fate has its gifts but it also has its drawbacks and challenges, many of which we can do something about.

For example, my mother and I were each filled with guilt and judged each other for not being better mothers or daughters. I was incapable of protecting my daughter from the dysfunction I inherited. We each suffered grief, loss, anger, sadness, and self-doubt.

We've expressed disappointment in each other and been our own harshest critics at times. I didn't understand why my mother stayed married to my father when he cheated on her chronically. My daughter didn't understand my divorcing her father. She vowed that she would never divorce or put her children through what I put her through.

And I sat powerless as she went through a painful divorce and was left to raise my first granddaughter on her own until she remarried. There is no doubt that if we knew how, we would have protected each other and tried to prevent suffering, but I'm not certain we loved ourselves enough to fully love each other.

Another reality I had to face was that when there are two daughters in a generation in our constellation, one sister is targeted, scorned, and despised while the other sister is brought up to take on, replicate, and deepen the psychosis. This happened with my grandmother and her daughters and with my mother and sister and me. When my sister joined ranks with Mom, for example, the dynamic was kept alive, which is how old patterns are passed along and travel forward into future generations.

No matter how much Mom was loved, she never had the love she craved from her own mother or my dad. Nothing else could make up for that loss. I realize now how unrequited and deeply dissatisfied she was with her lot in life while unwittingly assuring that she would pass her fate along to her own daughters.

I fear Mom carried regret, self-judgment, and pain to her grave. I vowed that would not be me. I think now of the assurances she sought from me in her final months—that I wasn't angry at her for being a bad mother, that Dad didn't hate her for leaving him alone in the ambulance the night he died.

Upon reflection, I think the anger she often felt was largely her own, built up over a lifetime of feeling unloved by her own mother. Forgiveness was unthinkable for her. Atonement was not in her vocabulary. I suspect she never felt worthy of all the love she did have in her life. It wasn't good enough. It didn't fill the emptiness she felt because she never heard the simple words "I love you" from her own mother.

Mom never understood why her mother didn't express love to her.

It haunted her. As a daughter in this line of women, I felt the same sorrow in my own life. I didn't understand what made me unlovable and unworthy of my mother's love.

I searched for a surrogate and found it in my grandmother. My daughter searched for a surrogate and found it in my mother. My granddaughter searched for a surrogate and found it in me. But each of us has had to learn a bitter lesson. We yearn for the understanding of our own mothers. We yearn for the unconditional love and their total acceptance of who we are and have become as women.

Over the years, I stood by and watched, feeling helpless, as resentment grew and each generation, in our own way, suffered from feelings of abandonment and ended up abandoning ourselves. The separations from each other that have been a part of our family dynamic isolate us from our mothers, from the source of love we seek yet at the same time often reject.

When I write about these dynamics now, they would seem unbelievable to me if not for the fact that I have lived this way for a good part of my life and passed on these unhealthy patterns. It's unthinkable that I would not dedicate the rest of my life to doing everything I can to shatter these illusions that have little or nothing to do with unconditional love.

I firmly believe that in some distant past generation of mothers and daughters in my line, love was the driving force. I hoped that at the end of my mother's life, she felt this kind of love for me and from me. I hope that was the beginning of a seismic shift in how women in my constellation will love each other and their daughters in the future.

Recently, I was sharing some of my discoveries about the impact of inherited trauma on my relationship with my daughter with one of my very closest friends. She lost her mother before her 40th birthday to cancer. When I told her about some issues my daughter and I were having, my friend said to me, "I don't understand. Do you have any idea what I would give to spend one more day with my Mom?"

I was reminded once again why it is so important that we don't allow some distant inherited trauma or pain to impact our relationships with our parents and children in the present. It is not easy to break the painful chains of inherited trauma, but when I think of the generations ahead and how the changes we make now may benefit them, I know it will be worth it in the end.

Learning to love, respect, and accept my mother as I have come to through introspection on both my successes and failures as a mother and daughter has changed me. All I can say is that I feel more at ease with who I am and more fully myself. The best I can do for my daughter and granddaughters with the rest of my life is to leave them a legacy of unconditional love and acceptance.

As we free ourselves from ancestral burdens whenever we see thoughts or actions influenced by the past and the hurt and trauma of old, we can fight our old conditioning. The challenge ahead as we bow to fate and move forward will surely be to deepen our ability to love unconditionally and throw off the lead-weighted winter coat of inherited trauma, broken bonds, and conditional love.

Mothers give life and the child receives it. That's one of the core tenets of Family Constellation Theory and its one of the most important truths I have learned in recent years. I wish I knew that a very long time ago. I hope that you can embrace these concepts now and find some understanding of yourself through your journey in inherited trauma.

What the future holds for any of us, how things improve for the better, is not for us to know at this moment in time. Our job is simply to allow for the possibilities and remain open. While inherited patterns may not jump off the page right now and illuminate what was fated to be in your life, I do have some suggestions that may help connect you to them.

When I first started studying Family Constellation Theory, I became fascinated with my ancestral line. I did a DNA test and then had some genealogical research done on my family line. I discovered more and more about the traumas that past generations in my family suffered, survived, and passed along. I wanted to know all that I could know. The dysfunctional pattern between the women in my family tracks back to at least my great-grandmother and likely beyond. It's freeing to know that these inherited traumas didn't start with you.

If you haven't done so, you might consider it. You might also want to encourage your own parents or grandparents to participate in DNA testing so that you can go back to prior generations. You might even consider making a gift of the test kits to family members.

Understanding my parents' roots helped me to better understand them and the people who they were. I only wish this technology had existed when my parents and grandparents were alive, but, instead, we are testing forward. In fact, my grandson and I still laugh at the unsurprising finding that we will never be sprinters or opera singers.

Your inquiries may even reunite you with relatives you never knew you had. My friend found an unknown first cousin who has since become an important part of her life, healing old traumas and teaching the family of the power of acceptance and unconditional love. The parallels in their personal stories were quite astounding.

What I've come to realize is how important it is that we leave a comprehensive family history for our own children and grandchildren, whether it's oral or written. Our traumas travel generationally through time, as do the blessings we receive. You may want to start chronicling the pieces of family history that you know, and that may help your family better understand the roots of family dysfunction, health factors, talents possessed, and opportunities seized.

Better yet, pick up the phone and call your parents or grandparents if they are alive. Make time to do something special with them or for them. Ask them the questions about their own lives or your grandparents that are on your mind. Don't take for granted that you still have the time.

CHAPTER 13

What We Really Feel

"Without forgiveness life is governed by ...
an endless cycle of resentment and retaliation."

—ROBERTO ASSAGIOLI

THROUGH THE TRAUMAS WE SUFFER AND BECAUSE OF THE INHERITED patterns of dysfunction that we may not even be aware of, we form emotional patterns and preferences that fit the roles we were destined to play within our family structure. Gaining an understanding of how your own predilections developed and why will allow you to move beyond them and expand your emotional range of expression appropriate to the situation you are in, if you choose to.

Emotional Preferences

Freeing ourselves from the past includes freeing ourselves emotionally. It may look different in each of our lives, but the psychological process is similar. We each have emotional preferences and at times the differences between us can separate us from the understanding and love we seek.

As we journey from trauma to healing, it is critical that we gain insight into our own emotional preferences, how they formed, and how to move beyond them constructively. In the process, we will learn how the emotional inclinations of others trigger automatic responses in us based upon the differences in our preferred emotions.

For example, my emotional preference was pain, and Mom's was anger, each of us having unconsciously developed a favored emotion in early childhood as a coping mechanism to survive familial dysfunction and trauma. Our choices later harmed our relationship. My mother ran from the pain she felt and I ran from the anger I felt.

This is how it works: Transmutation of emotions is a psychological process whereby we turn one or more emotions that we want to repress into another emotion that we can better cope with inside ourselves. My inclination has always been to turn my anger into hurt feelings, which I could better tolerate. My mother did the opposite. Consequently, we often ended up provoking each other and the feelings we each had buried.

I grew up with a sister who developed the same emotional preference as Mom. When I would hear them yell at each other and say hurtful things, I feared their encounters would turn into physical brawls. However, slamming doors, hanging up the phone, and throwing small objects were acceptable expressions of emotion. Angry outbursts didn't seem to faze them.

Anger, as I see it, has malignant and self-righteous elements that are meant to harm its targets. I always felt small or insignificant in comparison to them when they were lashing out. Early in my life, I realized that if I got angry back I'd be just like them. I didn't want to be anything like them. Whatever anger I might have felt, I promptly threw—figuratively speaking—into an incinerator, to burn and turn into ashes of pain I could tolerate.

Sitting here now, I wish I had allowed myself to feel my anger and express it.

I still remember the first therapist I had in graduate school asking if I felt angry about something my mother had done to me that I was recounting in a session. I adamantly denied that I even had any anger inside. "My mother and sister have a corner on that market. That's just not who I am," I said.

That wasn't true, of course, but at the time I sincerely believed it was. I had developed a real talent for transmuting even the hint of an angry sensation inside me into hurt feelings. Is that to say that I never acted out in anger? No, of course not. But it was rare that I let it show or that I lost control. I know that when I did, those around me took special notice. I could see them flinch and back away from me—not an effect I want to have on anyone.

When I continued to deny I had any anger, my therapist gave me exercises to do. I had to practice getting to my anger and letting it out in nondestructive ways. She suggested screaming in the shower or the car as I drove across the Golden Gate Bridge to attend classes or do supervised work at the counseling center.

She also had me pounding on pillows with a tennis racket until I felt my own anger rise. Those efforts weren't particularly successful, but I stayed with the process.

Emotional preference and expression often have their roots, as in my case, early in life and are influenced by inherited traumas and patterns. The angry person becomes the perpetrator. The person yelled at, bullied, or taunted becomes the victim. Some relationship systems are hopelessly caught up in the perpetrator-victim dynamics. No matter how we may attempt to change that cycle by staying in it and holding tight to those trauma-related attitudes, those attempts at transforming dysfunction may not be possible.

As Dr. Ruppert teaches, "The issue is about our own internal life becoming healthier. Individually and collectively, we need to work on our own psychological health." Finding ourselves doesn't harm other people, but it can help to alter our relationships in positive ways and break generational patterns.

We aren't working on our internal lives to change others but rather to heal ourselves. And yet, Ruppert adds, "It may, however, interfere with their impulse to abuse me for their trauma-survival strategies. But that could be a good opportunity for them to deal with their own traumas."

No Longer Afraid

Over the years that I have worked with hostile and volatile people in the course of my professional life, I have learned to manage their anger and rage. I learned how to cope with these behaviors in others but not how to express anger or feel it myself. And when anger is more personal and directed at me I retreat.

Why was it that I couldn't confront my sister or mother? I could sit across a conference room table with some of the most potentially frightening individuals I had ever met. During some of my encounters, I was working with people who were on the verge of physically harming others, but I was neither angry nor afraid.

In the mid-1990s, one of the first cases we handled through our new company, Confidante, Inc., stands out in my mind. Norm and I had been hired by a high-tech machine shop to conduct a threat assessment regarding the explosive behavior of one of their most highly skilled computerized lathe operators. The precipitating event was a serious argument that started in the breakroom and erupted into a physical fight in the parking lot after the shop closed. The loser of the fight filed a formal complaint with company management.

Norm drove to the worksite with me. The plan was that he would work with the company's CEO, general counsel, human resources, and administrative personnel. The goal for his day was to generate the information we would need to amend their policies and procedures and put them in compliance with current employment laws.

The plan for my day was that I would interview the complainants and do a threat assessment concerning the above-referenced accused. We both agreed that this confrontational personality type would not respond well to another man, most especially, an attorney.

What we didn't want to do was motivate him to any sort of inappropriately aggressive behavior. By the time I met with the employee of concern, Norm would be finished with his work and could position himself close enough to overhear our interactions and intervene if necessary. This was of great comfort to me.

When we got there, the machine shop manager and union representative were engaged in a contentious argument as to whether or not I would even be allowed to interview the accused. While the company was privately owned, it was a unionized environment and the parties involved disagreed about the need for an assessment. The union denied he was violent. To them, the company was overreacting and this was just "how the guys work things out in the shop. They take it out back."

However, according to the accused's supervisor, this latest incident was just one in a long string of increasingly dangerous confrontations. I was also told that the only reason he hadn't been fired was that he was an exceptionally talented machinist who turned out more work in less time than any other of their employees.

If this shouting match I was witnessing was the standard of conduct tolerated by management, I thought, I dreaded the hostility I would face in the workforce. It was only after speaking with the union rep that he confided his own fear to me regarding the employee. He decided to allow me to interview coworkers and, finally, the threatening party himself.

I told the supervisor I would like to see the working environment before settling into the small office where I would be conducting the interviews. He took me up a flight of stairs to a window where I could take a look at the entire operation. I was surprised by the noise level and to see how many sparks were flying around from steel-cutting equipment, torches, and arc welders. Men were shouting; forklifts were moving back and forth.

My first interviews were with the employee's coworkers. They were genuinely fearful that the rage-filled behavior of this individual and the fistfight that he started after work two days prior was a step too far. "Charlie the Brooding Giant," as they called him, had lost control and they didn't want to work with him anymore.

The machine shop, they said, was filled with tools that could be and had been used to settle disagreements and fights in the past. Several interviewees also reported that Charlie carried a handgun in the glove compartment of his truck and they anticipated a day when the mounting tension in the shop would push him over the brink. They feared the day he would enter the shop "guns a-blazing." And trust me when I tell you I was more than a little afraid that this might be that day.

The center of this particular storm was a burly, bearded machinist, whose mere appearance was frightening, his demeanor ominous. To see him was to fear him, but I smiled as Charlie entered the room. I'm not sure how I managed to do that or how convincing I was.

It was one thing to have come into the Pettit & Martin workplace after the violence ended. It was a totally different experience to sit across from an individual with a proven propensity for violence.

Charlie wasn't one for introductions and pleasantries. I don't think he really cared who I was and what we were doing there. When I started asking questions, his answers were long-winded angry rants. There didn't seem to be anybody or anything safe from Charlie's rage and no one who hadn't wronged him in some way. Even the union rep who was fighting to protect his job and stop the threat assessment was a target of his wrath. From Charlie's own description of a typical day in his life, I learned that he woke up angry and went to bed angry. He described how often he screamed and swore at his television when something was broadcasted that upset him.

When Charlie started complaining about drivers who shared the roadways with him, his fists began to soundly thump the metal. He was, from my point of view, one more road-rage incident away from turning deadly violent, and I was close to ending the interview.

The personnel records that we reviewed confirmed that Charlie was often the target of complaints by his coworkers. But he also complained often about his coworkers and the conditions in the workplace. Overall, the records confirmed that the culture in this workplace was abysmal. They included complaints of yelling, swearing, and tampering with coworkers' private property and tools. There were also reports of physical altercations and disagreements that were not resolved by management.

It wasn't that Charlie was some disgruntled, calculated would-be workplace shooter, but he was indeed a powder keg with a very short fuse. Angry emotions at this level of intensity lack rationality, and the person feeling them loses control. Charlie was a classic bully, and I needed to find out what fueled his anger.

The buttons on his coveralls were open to just above his waist and his massive, hairy chest heaved as the sheer volume of angry words poured out. There was a long, thick gold chain that hung around Charlie's neck. It was as incongruous as it could be with his overall demeanor. It seemed to bounce and swing, flashing light with each angry expulsion of air. The effect, to my surprise, was mildly hypnotizing. I listened patiently as his tirade continued for over an hour until he seemed to exhaust himself. I think the saving grace for me was that his anger was not personal to me.

As the flow of his words slowed, I sensed that he was curious about what I was thinking. He was likely wondering how I was able to sit for so long and let him rage on about everything and anything he wanted. For the first time, he began to talk to me rather than at me.

He said, "So you think I'm some crazy workplace shooter? What do you think, doc? You're the pro. Everyone else is afraid of me, why not you?" When I didn't answer immediately, he added, "Hey, doc, what you got to say for yourself?" Charlie leaned across the table and I sat back in my chair. How I responded next was wholly unexpected even to me but absolutely reflected what I was thinking.

I said, "Charlie, what I think is that it must be hard to be you, walking around with all that anger and rage every day all day. Wherever you go, whatever you do, whoever you're with, there you are. Whatever else you might feel, or may have felt at one time, you've spun into anger. I just keep thinking about how hard it would be to be you." I told him, "And, Charlie, that's so damn sad."

Charlie's breathing slowed, the gold chain lay still and he released a sigh of exhaustion that had been buried deep. Then an amazing thing happened. His eyes began to moisten, tears formed in the corners of his eyes and fell, rolling slowly down his face and onto his chest. He began wiping away the tears with the back of his huge hands.

The anger that filled him visibly dissolved. Silence surrounded us for the first time since we sat down together. When he began to speak, it was in a softer, almost childlike voice. Charlie said, "I haven't cried since I was six years old, but I feel like you've seen me, I mean, the real me. Nobody has ever seen me in my family. They were angrier than me so I figured I had to be madder than them and then people would notice."

"That's an easy conclusion to reach as a kid, Charlie, but I don't think it's working for you now."

Somehow, I had been able to sit there in the middle of his rage. I stepped into his shoes to try and grasp what it must have been like to be Charlie. I couldn't know that my honest reaction was something he had been craving for most of his life. I gave him a safe place to fall that day where he was able to release the pain buried under his rage.

Anyone else who might have told him the truth had been driven away years before. He didn't want to shoot anybody. He didn't want to fight and he didn't want to run over anybody with his truck. He didn't want people to fear him and he did not want to lose his job.

What Charlie did want was someone to recognize and relate to the wounded child hidden under all that anger. He seemed exhausted by the perpetrator role he had perfected over the years, with his aggressive, short-tempered attitude that had alienated him from coworkers, friends, and family.

I can't tell you where all his anger and rage came from or whether the reasons for it were justified or caused by an abusive early life. But I do know that both our lives changed that day.

Charlie did not have to continue to transmute all of his pain and unrequited love into anger. Together, we had a breakthrough, and he was able to step back from the brink of disaster. I came away with renewed hope. There are people who are redeemable, and nobody had to die.

While it's true that there are evil, sick people in the world who commit unthinkable acts, the majority of individuals that threaten to kill themselves or others in places where they work do not want to make good on their threats. It's often a wakeup call to them of how far they have fallen and how exposed they have become.

At the same time, we can't risk ignoring people like Charlie. We can't stand by as their behavior gets more and more outrageous and they push themselves into dark corners. When that's allowed to happen, they see no escape other than violence to themselves or others.

While I will never accept that Dad's murder was anything other than an act of pure evil, I hadn't lost sight of the fact that there are many people like Charlie who just want to be seen.

No matter what approach I took with my own sister, I would never get her to listen to me or have a breakthrough. I was not the one that would cause her tears to fall or her pain to come through. We had our predestined roles, our preferred emotions and well-established patterns, such as I have described with the generations of women in my line. As long as she continued to live out our generational inheritance, I would never change the relationship or her feelings about me. I was not someone she could love. That would threaten her very existence. I would not be the one from whom she could accept love or give forgiveness.

What I learned that day with Charlie—what I came to terms with— was that I had enough of the old pattern in my family. No matter how many times I banged my head up against the wall of defense my sister had erected around herself, I would never make a dent in her armor.

I don't know if you call that giving up or letting go—maybe a little of both. What I would say is that I had learned enough about my own emotional nature to understand why I do many of the things that I do and to change and eliminate what I no longer was willing to do.

Beyond the confines of limited emotional constructs, we can increase our emotional intelligence and increase our capacity to recognize our feelings and those of others without automatically responding as we were once conditioned to do. We can learn to identify feelings and discern between them. Am I really hurt, or am I actually angry but afraid to express my true feelings?

I hope that you will explore your own emotional nature and preferences and find the courage to break free of the perpetrator-victim cycles that formed so you could survive the drama and traumas you have experienced. Try reflecting on how you feel right now. Simply name the feeling or make a list of your changing emotions throughout the day. In the evening, look back at the emotions you listed during the day. Explore the context or circumstances in which these emotions arose. What ratio of positive to negative emotions do you have on any given day? Which dominate and what triggers your different feeling states?

Just doing a simple practice like this can help. You will more easily recognize your own emotional preferences, how they were selected, and where they originated. This will allow you to work on changing the triggers and reducing the negative emotions by stopping them when they arise. First comes the awareness and with it the power to change old, largely automatic patterns.

We can over time use emotional information to inform our thinking and behavior and adapt to the situation and circumstances we are in to achieve our goals. We can learn to monitor our feelings rather than repress them. We can learn to express them in healthy ways that can improve our relationships rather than harm them.

We can also learn to differentiate between safe and unsafe relationships so that we recognize and can walk away from those people in our lives who are, for whatever reason, hopelessly caught in the grip of the victim-perpetrator cycle. We can wish them well but free ourselves.

CHAPTER 14

Turning Obstacles
into Gifts

"Family Constellations transforms the family burdens to blessings.
Unconscious love becomes Conscious love."

—BERT HELLINGER

I HOPE I'VE INSPIRED YOU TO DIG DEEP, REFLECT ON YOUR LIFE'S lessons, and find practical ways to apply them to make positive change. Don't let the traumas of your life define or limit you. Choose your own future amid the limitless possibilities that exist beyond the boundaries of inherited suffering and family dysfunction.

I would love to tell you that there is some final "there" to be found. I can't. The path through our lives—the journey from trauma to survival to healing—has its moments. The more truthful we are with ourselves, the more we understand that we will have our instances of great insight, understanding, and peace. We also realize that something, internal or external, will come along to upset our newfound balance but that we will be better prepared to respond to it and return to our safe places to fall.

The Gift of Fate

It's been several years since I bowed to fate and embraced the women who preceded me in my ancestry line. When I look back over the years, I can see the energy and pain that went into trying to make my past something other than what it was. And yet everything and everyone in my life had been laid out just as fate intended.

I yearned for a different mother or a big sister that acted like a sister. I wished I had not lost my father when or how I did. But on one fine day while on a retreat in Sedona, Arizona, in 2015, I gave up wishing my life was not my life. I experienced my fate and ancestors in a new way. I was humbled by the powerful forces that had shaped me before I was even born.

I found the unconditional love inside myself that I had been looking for and hoping to find in the women in my line. I stopped longing for what never was or would be. I was free from the chains that tethered me to the past. I felt that the world was my stage and I was the capable playwright. I had the ability to perfect loving roles for those who traveled through my life and those who stayed.

I'm not implying that life has been a breeze since then or that I have been free from doubt, pain, or heartache. But I can say that I am facing my life and its challenges from a solid foundation of self-love, understanding, and acceptance. I see options that I hadn't seen before. I see what I can do differently. I look at the choices of the women in my generation and beyond—my sister, my daughter, and my granddaughters.

I make choices that I believe strengthen the foundation of uncon-ditional love and free will for me and, I hope, for my daughter and granddaughters. I've reaped the rewards; I've seen indications that they have, too, as I continue to detach from unconscious choices and patterns of old. In the process, obstacles became gifts and tools that I could apply to what I learned.

In Family Constellation Theory, Dr. Hellinger has been quoted as saying that he believes our lives follow a "script, a hidden plan from the beginning and, therefore, we can compare it to a film which follows a screenplay in every detail and determines how it ends."

It may be true that my fate was largely predetermined and that people and events that occurred were meant to be. I am also confident that I have free will and the ability to choose what to do each time fate comes knocking. Implicit in free will is saying yes to something and no to something else.

When I said, "Yes, this is my fate, this is my inheritance. I see how it is," I also said, "I accept it, and moving forward I choose a different path." It's been several years since then and my journey continues. Every day, in some small way, I say yes to what makes me feel more alive and no to whatever makes me feel less alive.

Walking in my fate I found my true self. I found the love within that had not been distorted almost beyond recognition and whose flow had survived generations of dysfunction, jealousy, anger, and conditional love. In our essence, I believe, there is beauty and the potential for greatness. What a different world we would live in today if all of us could touch that truth and live it, if we were willing to search inside ourselves and find the unconditional love that so often lies buried in the ruins of trauma, missed opportunity, and familial entanglements. Under the rubble lives our true and best nature.

I take a Sedona journey annually. In a supremely spiritual place in Boynton Canyon, I found all the safety I needed to plumb the depths of my past and free myself from dysfunctional patterns and people that are not supportive or understanding of the changes I have made.

One day at a spa outside Sedona where I stay on my healing adventures, I sat at the smoothie bar alone. A gentle wind was blowing between the canyon walls, and the sun beamed down. The pine trees clung vertically to the red rocks. The world seemed to be in order and at peace.

Somehow, the storms and conditions I had weathered brought me to this moment. The circumstances of my life seemed less important and traumatic now. I came to the realization that there was no truth I needed to defend or protect myself from anymore. I was content with myself as I listened to the ancient sound of a Native American wood flute drifting in from the lounge.

Behind the bar was a woman named Maura, according to her name tag. She was likely 20 years younger than me—my daughter's age. We started chatting and I found out she was from San Francisco. Maura started talking about growing up in Pacific Heights and attending Marin Country Day School.

The Clay Street house I lived in was in the same neighborhood where she grew up, and my own kids went to Marin Country Day School. The more we talked, the more we had in common. Then, Maura started talking about how San Francisco began to change when she was a young teen. She said, "The city wasn't safe anymore. We couldn't walk the streets alone."

"I had the same experience," I said.

Maura nodded her head in understanding. She said, "Bad people started coming into Pacific Heights. It had always been a safe neighborhood. The final straw for me and my family was when a nice man was walking his dog with his wife. They were robbed. The man got shot and killed on Maple Street." I confess my jaw dropped.

She continued, "We lived only two blocks away from where it happened. I will never forget that night. We could hear all the sirens. My parents locked all the doors and turned out the lights. We were terrified."

Before responding, I took a sip of my green smoothie to give me time to find the right words for this moment. "Maura, it was my father that was killed that night."

She gasped and came around from behind the bar and hugged me tightly. Here we were, in one of the most serene places on earth, surrounded by beauty, remembering the most terrifying night of my life and the event that robbed both of us of the only home either of us had known, San Francisco.

It was quite an unexpected exchange, but, I reminded myself, this is the Sedona way. I couldn't think of a better place to be reminded of this life-altering loss or the small miracles that occurred here. Maura unexpectedly gave me a gift. Dad's life and loss changed the life of a perfect stranger, seemingly for the better. And she never forgot. Dad was remembered. His death mattered.

It was a moment of insight for me. I didn't fall into the trauma of my loss or Dad's murder. I was actually grateful. It was a reminder of the man who made my life possible and worth living. This chance meeting was validation that healing had taken hold of me and violence had lost its grip.

I was living the life I always wanted. I had more positive influences than negative, and the scales of justice had turned in my favor. With my mother gone and my siblings out of my life, I was on my own in a great new way.

Stepping out of your life for a time, touching the deepest levels of the innately human, unconditional love that exists in all of us and breaking new ground for the future—wherever this happens, it can be a universal phenomenon buried and seemingly forgotten in broken psyches of individuals and the divided and often hateful world of today. I am fortunate. I found a safe place to fall. Will you take the time and make the effort to find the beauty that lies within you and is reflected in the eyes of those who love you unconditionally?

It saddens me to have crossed paths with many people who are so overwhelmed or consumed by the challenges of their fate that they turn on each other rather than search within themselves or reject a helping hand when it is extended in peace. I watch as some people skate across the ice, slipping and sliding through life without the fulfillment and joy that I know can be found.

I am grateful that I bowed to fate while also saying, "No, I will not breathe new life into the hardships I inherited or limit the possibilities to excel that exist for me." I simply cannot knowingly choose to continue to reinjure myself or those I love. Can you?

My life could have gone in many different directions. I have traveled roads that were dead ends. Often, I had to double back and retrace my steps because the road I was on didn't lead me where I wanted to go or took me away from myself and my goals. As I integrate the challenges I have confronted, I am walking down a beautiful new path.

As Dr. Assagioli famously said about life, "There is no certainty; there is only adventure." It is because of this truism that I am inspired to live fully, love completely, give freely, and learn until the end. At this moment, as I sit on the couch in my living room, it's very quiet inside me. I smile at the thought that you, too, will embrace your life as the grand adventure that it is.

For now, I am surrounded by the sound of the rain on the skylight overhead and the music of the chimes singing in the wind. I watch as the leaves of the oaks and sycamores sway to a rhythm familiar only to them. The glowing embers in the fireplace give off warmth. I have found the perfect backdrop for discovery and new adventures. At the same time, I understand that our moods change as the weather does. Either shift can set us on a new adventure, even when we are perfectly content with where we are.

A Predictable Storm

Like the weather, the flow of inner life has a way of changing on us. It's important not to let the changes distract us from our ultimate goal of improving our life experiences. Order turns to chaos before returning to order once again. For example, one recent morning I woke up and my mood was sunny, bright, and relaxed. All was in order, or so I thought.

I intended to write a new segment of this book. While enjoying my morning coffee ritual, I turned on the local news. I heard the meteorologist explain that this day was going to be a very wet one. In fact, she described it as "an atmospheric river of concentrated moisture."

And right when the Doppler said the storm would arrive, it did, and it came in with a vengeance. I was reminded at that moment how vulnerable we are to outside forces while still being able to maintain the locus of control within ourselves. At least, I hoped that was true.

At the time, I also had an inner storm brewing as a result of some intense research and exploration of human nature I had completed the day before. I was experiencing my own turmoil and seeking a safe place to fall. So, I lit a fire in the fireplace and sat down to write.

Dark thoughts were gathering like ominous clouds threatening my peace of mind. Reading through some of my old journals, I was thrown into a past I thought I had dealt with and left behind. Without warning, I became that little girl in her tiny room in the corner of the big house, alone and afraid, waiting for Daddy to come home.

I felt at the mercy of an angry sister and mother. My very survival felt threatened. I was the victim again, and they were my adversaries. In my memory, the victim-perpetrator cycle was activated.

I realized then that I could be pulled back into the inherited trauma of the women in my line. Or I could hold firm to all that I learned, yearned for, and gained. I asked myself how I could, in good conscience, plunge myself back into the turmoil from which I had only recently escaped.

I wished those memories away, but it wasn't as easy as saying, *be gone.* I wondered if there comes a time for each of us when we have stirred up and relived past traumas and dysfunction sufficiently enough that we are free to move on without reliving it yet again. I hoped this was that time.

In the tree-covered hills that surround my house, I watched carefully as the already saturated earth continued to absorb the downpour of rain. Hopefully, the deep-rooted trees could maintain their footing and keep from sliding down the hill. I was facing a similar challenge inside myself.

I wondered how many storms of my own psychodrama I could absorb and how many of them I needed to rehash in my mind. Generations past, present, and future collided inside me and threatened to pull me down as I, like the trees outside, held firm against the pressure.

The old patterns of behavior and ineffective coping mechanisms were waking up and attempting to lure me into familiar ways of being no matter how many times they failed me in the past. But I was reminded, too, of the new patterns that had been evolving that had proven to be successful in strengthening and helping me become the person I am today. Order and chaos were in a standoff.

The pulls from the past are powerful and don't want to be ignored, but I have found the will to resist temptation and reject the opportunity to revert to old mechanisms. This was just another opportunity to do so, I told myself. I knew, too, that there would be similar challenges on the path ahead, no matter how far I traveled.

So there I sat, on one of the stormiest days of the year. The wind was tearing at the trees as the rain was whipping at the windows. I was intent on calming myself. I pondered the questions that moved like storm clouds through my mind.

I asked myself, "How do I spread out my wings far enough, open my heart wide enough, and suspend judgment long enough to hold the order and disorder that exists—the contradictions, the good and the bad, the old and the new, the traumas and the healing?"

If I posed that same question to you, how would you answer me? Can you recall a time when order turned to chaos in your world? Do you know how you were able to find order out of disorder? Were you able to stabilize yourself, or did you need help? This is a worthwhile conversation to have with yourself. You may even want to pull out your journal and take some notes. When you feel lost, your own wisdom and experience may guide you back to a safe place.

That day, I was able to recover calm and order for myself. The trials and tribulations are real. I can touch them and feel them. I feel like my ancestors reached back through time that stormy day and begged me, "Don't abandon us. Don't reject our fate. We left it for you."

It was unsettling that a part of me still answered their call and was trying to drag me into the past. I closed my eyes and reminded myself that my journey requires compassion, unconditional love, patience, and acceptance—my own.

By mid-afternoon, both storms had passed and I was at peace. The past will always dwell inside me, but I don't need to allow it to take over the future. Order returned and safe spaces held firm, inside and out. The next time you find a storm gathering inside of yourself, I trust that you will find the strength to weather it and learn from it.

PART V

Your Future Is in Your Hands

CHAPTER 15

Making Peace with the Past

"Resistance is loyalty to the old and prevents development. Every expectation is thus linked to something already known. Only what shakes me to the core leads me onward. The rigidity breaks, growth follows. In the end we can only marvel at where we find ourselves.

—Bert Hellinger

I trust that you would like nothing more than to free yourself from the harm of trauma and the influence that its remnants have on you still. How do you plan to turn the corner? How will you resist the pull from the past and move beyond a stressed and traumatized psyche to embrace a healthier state of mind?

Dr. Ruppert warns us that we have to avoid being pulled back into the very victim-perpetrator cycle we are turning away from if we are to walk a more fulfilling, life-sustaining path. At times, the temptation is great and the forces of fate, family, and nature are powerful. We need to resist the temptation. More often than not, it is our own fear we have to move beyond. We must name it to face it and free ourselves from it.

To quote Dr. Ruppert, "We are afraid that, if we do break the cycle, we will be lonely and subjected to accusations and guilt from those who themselves do not dare to exit. Here it is of enormous importance to recognize perpetrator and victim attitudes in ourselves and others."

By so doing, we will be able to better recognize whether those around us are acting out of their healthy psychological parts, love us unconditionally, and appreciate our journey toward healthier ways of being. Or we may discover that they are more interested in our remaining within the circle of codependency to keep the victim-perpetrator dynamic alive. We may be ready to break free while they may resist our efforts or reject us. They may find safety within the familiar yet unhealthy dynamics.

Personally, I had no illusions about the harmful nature of the conditional love and dysfunctional relationships in my family or my need to break free. I was moving beyond the trauma I had experienced. At the same time, I wanted to make peace with my mother and relate to her in a way that was healthy for both of us.

I did not want to slip into either the victim or perpetrator role. I wanted to exercise my new ability to love unconditionally, putting pain and bitterness aside. I knew I would be testing myself and my resolve. Neutralizing the negative relationship patterns we had been in together would be difficult.

I believed we still had time to come to terms with the ghosts that had haunted our relationship all my life. I was open to doing so because, in part, of the gentle yet persistent urgings of Norm. I learned from him that growing up with unconditional love helps you understand the emotions of others and how they love.

There is something very healing about being able to give unconditional love to someone who has never had it and, consequently, couldn't give it. Have you had that gratifying experience? I had learned to give that kind of love. I knew I would forever regret it if I didn't find a way to accept my mother, better understand her, and love her unconditionally before she died.

The older I got the more I treasured the life I had been given. I knew the self-harm I would be doing if I continued to reject the very person that gave me the gift of life. I didn't know how much time Mom and I would have to heal.

When it got really hard and giving up was on my mind, it was Norm's perseverance and patience that kept me going. He never gave up on me. I came to accept that the extended life of my mother was providing me with the opportunity I needed to heal the break in my bond with her before her death.

As Mom's life lingered on, my fear of rejection weakened and withered even as she did. With her 100th birthday approaching, I didn't want to tempt fate by waiting to say what I needed to say or waiting to hear what I needed to hear. But it wasn't until years later that I came to fully appreciate just how significant this process of forgiveness and atonement was to my own journey.

According to Dr. Hellinger's Family Constellation Theory, there is no relationship more connected to our life, our wholeness, happiness, and success than our relationship with our mothers. He contends that our mothers are literally "the fountain of life."

Mothers give life and children receive life. That is the birth order—mothers give and children receive. I hope you were blessed with an unconditionally loving mother and can embrace the gift that is and the advantage that can give you over your lifetime. Without it, there is an emptiness that is difficult to fill but critical to healing.

Mom deserved my unconditional love. I couldn't think of a more fruitful relationship and opportunity to live what I had learned. If I rejected her now, I would be rejecting part of myself and the life I had learned to love. I also came to understand that accepting myself and my life gave me the capacity to accept Mom.

I knew that if I continued to judge my mother and her love for me, I risked that she would die having reservations about me. I did not want that. The quality of my relationship with her had troubled me for much of my life. It shaped me in ways seen and unseen, conscious and unconscious.

Our early relationship determined our feelings about each other and our behavior toward each other over the rest of our lives. I carried with me the pain of separation from her and a sense of being lost and unloved. Feeling rejected, I rejected her so she would feel the pain I felt.

Even when she was there for me, my self-rejection remained. I couldn't embrace her or accept the love she had to give. I needed to change that. I couldn't let her life and our relationship end the way it began.

Expressions of Unconditional Love

In the years since Mom's death, I was so grateful that I was able to forgive and love her unconditionally. There is nothing I can think of that I wanted to say but didn't. I hope that, if she were here, she would say the same.

I think the saddest thing is to die or watch someone you love die with regret for what they did or didn't do. To me, it is a gift to have the time to say our goodbyes and move beyond traumas that we too often avoid talking about.

Whether it's fear of causing more pain, fear of rejection, or anger and resentment that stops us from forgiveness and atonement, it seems irrelevant the longer I live. I often wonder what it is we are defending ourselves from and why we hold onto those thoughts and feelings that keep us from healing.

With my mother, the power of love overcame the pain and we were able to heal old wounds. We shared forgiveness and made peace that we never had before during her final years. I learned to love Mom unconditionally and accept the love she had to give.

I came to realize just how toxic the withholding of forgiveness is and how powerful and purifying forgiveness can be. Forgiving my mother did not mean accepting past behavior, but it did mean letting go. Why would we hold onto some bitterness we wish we never felt in the first place? Why would we continue to reinjure ourselves and trap ourselves in the trauma of the perpetrator-victim cycle? I knew I wasn't going to.

I visited Mom frequently in those days. I would stop for her favorite orchids and loved that she displayed them in the little den in a place of honor on the wooden oriental chest. It now sits in my office as a reminder of the later, better years. We shared precious time together, often just the two of us. Sometimes my kids and grandchildren came with me; at other times, my brother or Norm came with me.

When Norm was with me, he would praise the power of my work and my success. Whenever the television media phoned and asked if I would come in to be interviewed concerning breaking workplace violence news, he would call Mom. Norm would advise her to tune in and Mom always did.

He wanted to make certain Mom shared his pride and knew that I was strong and successful. He told her how much I loved her. Mom would stare at him and shake her head in affirmation as he talked. I felt that she developed a new respect for me. It felt wonderful to have someone on my side to balance out the lopsided reality of my family's power structure and the negativity that had undermined my relationship with her.

I could see that the unconditional love Mom felt coming from me softened her heart, that, in those days, was heavy with guilt, regret, and remorse. We never had another ugly moment and there were many gifts in those days. I was able to tell Mom my truth. Instead of rejection, acceptance filled our reunion.

She expressed her love to me more often and genuinely in those years than ever before. I stopped questioning whether she loved me or not. I now was certain that she did. She was not as negative as she once was. Gratefully, I was able to be more open and less defensive with her. I felt safe and respected by her.

Mom confessed her fears and regrets to me. We had long discussions about death and dying. She apologized to me for all the ways she couldn't give to me over the years. We spoke openly of the pain of my father's infidelities and she giggled when she told me she almost had an affair once herself.

Although Mom lacked psychological astuteness, in her own way, she expressed her regret for showing favoritism and not expressing her love more. Unknown to her, she had repeated the hurtful legacy that she had inherited from her mother and passed on to me.

She shared with me that not once in her life had her mother told her she loved her. My heart ached for her. Mom appeared to be so child-like, still craving the love of her mother that she never felt. I learned that Mom never felt loved and always believed she was less than her sister, Hannah, who was my grandmother's clear favorite.

This was evidenced in one final vindictive statement in the division of my grandmother's estate. And because of this, my mother told me, she would never give in to my sister's unrelenting pressure to cut me out of her will. All the thoughts that haunted Mom as she approached death, she shared openly.

When Mom asked me one day if I thought Dad forgave her for not getting into the ambulance with him that fateful night, I assured her that he already had. At other times, we would talk of that night so long ago, the trauma of which she would carry heavily with her to her grave. She struggled alone with the guilt that many survivors experience. On the outside, though, the way she lived and enjoyed her life, you never would have thought she had suffered so. She was just better at covering it up than others.

Looking back, I know that our best times were the rare stretches when we were alone together and there was no interference or complicating factors. It just took us longer to find common ground and to navigate past the people and events that drove us apart. I believe most people in our lives thought that our relationship was beyond repair, but they were wrong.

It was, after all, an inherited pattern for mothers and daughters to be at odds in our family. Who would have thought I would be able to heal this lineage? I would have deeply regretted it if we hadn't tried one more time and succeeded.

In retrospect, I think the greatest gift I gave to my mother was the life I gave to my own children and the life they gave to theirs. They exchanged the love and compatibility with Mom that I didn't, and I love them more than they will ever know for the joy they gave her. They took a burden off of my shoulders that had become too heavy to carry and completed a continuous circle of love. And they gave me hope that we could break the dysfunctional patterns that seemed generations in the making.

Is there someone somewhere who you hold yourself back from fully loving or forgiving? Do you harbor ill will toward yourself or have regrets for deeds done or left undone? This is a good time to reflect and make a list of regrets along with a plan for remedying them. Then you can create the opportunity to live the rest of your life without collecting any new ones. Perhaps you will discover love where you had given up hope of finding it.

This is an opportunity to have an honest conversation with yourself about unfinished business you may have with those you love or some way in which you find it difficult to forgive and love yourself. Healing happens from within and nourishes the heart.

A friend recently reminded me of a quote from Eleanor Roosevelt that I want to offer you: "Yesterday is history, tomorrow is a mystery, and today is a gift." Take this thought with you into your safe place to fall, which I hope by now is well established within and around you. I hope you are able to make peace with your path and embrace those who make your life worth celebrating.

CHAPTER 16

The Possibilities Are Limitless

*"Age helps one to acquire some of the perspectives necessary
to create harmony among apparent contradictions."*

—Roberto Assagioli

There is no pinnacle of peace or threshold of understanding
that doesn't get challenged when we are healing from trauma. We
add unnecessary stress to already stressful circumstances. Recovery
seems elusive and healing is difficult. Our nervous system responds
to the world around us by going into survival mode, leaving our
healthy psyche out of reach.

The work of Dr. Dan Siegel, clinical professor of psychiatry at
UCLA School of Medicine and executive director of the Mindsight
Institute, immediately comes to mind. He first coined the term
"window of tolerance" that is widely used to describe the optimal
level of functioning for people.

After a trauma, however, the human window of tolerance is nar-
rowed dramatically and we are forced to operate outside any healthy
zone. Our emotions are often intense and difficult to manage. Our
capacity to think rationally is greatly diminished, and our mental
health suffers. We vacillate between feeling overwhelmed and shutting down.

When we are within our own window of tolerance, we are generally able to process and integrate information despite the pressures we face. From there, we can respond to the demands of everyday life without much difficulty; we can thrive. It's different for everyone. Some of us operate in a wider or narrower zone than others, and our zones change at different times within our own lives.

Simply put, within the window of tolerance, your brain is functioning well and can effectively process the stimuli you are exposed to. This affords you the possibility to self-reflect, think rationally about the situation you are in, and make sound decisions. We can learn to manage stressful situations without our level of functioning suffering.

This complex mental process can be useful to grasp. It offers a way to identify our own ideal zone for functioning and find our way back to it when we are in trouble. See whether the following diagram helps you apply the concept to your own experiences.

There are also many self-soothing practices that you can include in your own healing process, such as mindfulness meditation, grounding strategies, deep-breathing exercises, use of positive affirmations, and self-talk.

Mindfulness is the practice of bringing our attention and awareness to the present. It allows us to pay attention to our thoughts, emotions, and physical feelings as they are occurring and adopt an attitude of acceptance to them. The practice relates to our window of tolerance. We learn in mindfulness exercises to regulate our emotions and not act on them irrationally. Similarly, using mindfulness, we can train ourselves to recognize where we are and what our best course of action is.

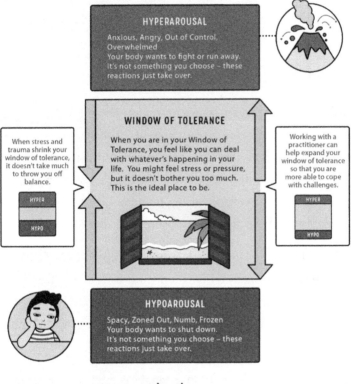

How Trauma Can Affect Your Window Of Tolerance

HYPERAROUSAL

Anxious, Angry, Out of Control, Overwhelmed
Your body wants to fight or run away.
It's not something you choose – these reactions just take over.

WINDOW OF TOLERANCE

When you are in your Window of Tolerance, you feel like you can deal with whatever's happening in your life. You might feel stress or pressure, but it doesn't bother you too much. This is the ideal place to be.

When stress and trauma shrink your window of tolerance, it doesn't take much to throw you off balance.

HYPER
HYPO

Working with a practitioner can help expand your window of tolerance so that you are more able to cope with challenges.

HYPER
HYPO

HYPOAROUSAL

Spacy, Zoned Out, Numb, Frozen
Your body wants to shut down.
It's not something you choose – these reactions just take over.

nicabm
© 2019 The National Institute for the Clinical Application of Behavioral Medicine

Grounding skills are also helpful in expanding the window of tolerance when stress causes you to fall outside of it. They can be as simple as pausing to take a deep breath and extending your exhale, taking a brief walk, adjusting your posture and standing tall, listening to a song you enjoy, or calling a friend you trust.

There are many books and websites that focus on mindfulness techniques and theories that can assist you on your journey. You can widen your own window of tolerance. The next time your comfort or safety is threatened by the challenges of life, you may find you have a broader perspective and an increased ability to respond.

Turning Trauma Around

I've done my best to learn from each trauma I have faced and expand my window of tolerance. In late June of 2014, I survived my own near-death experience from a raging infection that left me hospitalized for five days, within a week of my mother's funeral. My doctors attributed the near-collapse of my immune system to the "perfect storm" of stress I experienced just before and after Mom's death.

I suffered from the same infection that had proven to be fatal to my maternal grandmother. As I fought my way back to health and when I felt safe again, I thought often of her. The right antibiotics, sound medical care, lots of love, and the will to live saved my life, but for my grandmother, by the time she was hospitalized, it was too late.

Dr. Hellinger would say, from a family constellation perspective, that almost repeating my grandmother's fate by dying at the hands of the same infection that killed her was a way to keep our generational bond alive. For me, the discovery of my own experiences being rooted in my ancestors has been freeing, even if at times it was also terrifying. Maybe I saved myself from my grandma's fate. Maybe I even broke the cycle for my own granddaughters.

Looking back, I don't know how I could have engaged in the deep psychological journey I have been on if I didn't have the time to be with myself. The journey would not have mattered without the time and space to digest and integrate each new discovery. My comfort with myself—my sense of safety—is serving me now, but there have been times along the way when I've been lonely.

It was difficult to step away from the roles I had played and the dynamics of familial dysfunction. I have faced rejection from people whom I love very much and who were not ready to break the victim-perpetrator cycle that can trap some of us for a lifetime.

My life now is largely free of drama. Even my work has shifted, and we are able to engage in more positive circumstances and people who want to grow and expand. The family relationships that have drawn closer are richer and more rewarding. Those closest to me remind me of the high price I once paid to maintain hurtful and unfulfilling relationships. The time I spend alone is largely peaceful, productive, and creative time. Life is more fluid and spontaneous. I am free to roam the far corners of my mind and uncover the parts of me that have long been silenced. I am no longer afraid of what I might find.

I accept that life isn't perfect. I don't mind having myself for company anymore. Perhaps I've been building the most important relationship any of us can cultivate—the one we have with ourselves. Reconciling with the past and moving forward has also meant leaving behind coping mechanisms and roles that no longer serve me.

A Place for Closure

On the anniversary of my father's death last year, I decided to return for the first time to the place where I sought solace all those years ago when I didn't even believe there was a future for me. I bundled up and drove across the Golden Gate Bridge. I made my way around the eucalyptus-lined road of the Presidio to park at Baker's Beach.

It was a late-November afternoon, darkened by a fog. I stood on the same spot on the wet sand as I had that earlier time when I implored him to appear, but now he felt like my shadow, always near.

I looked up at the house on the hill where my mother was born. "I'm okay," I told my long-gone Grandpa Garrett. A blast from a foghorn answered me.

I began a slow walk down the abandoned stretch of beach. It was Dad I was here to talk to and my life I was here to celebrate with him. "Oh, Dad, where do I even begin?" I said. "It's been 43 years almost to the day since I lost you."

The wind picked up a little, carrying my words out to sea or maybe up to the sky so Dad could hear. Then I told him everything: the realizations I'd made, the hard work I'd done, the clarity and healing I'd gained sorting through childhood trauma and the impact and aftermath of his death—I shared it all. I looked up and was surprised to find that I had walked the length of the shoreline. I turned and looked at the sea. I could have sworn I heard the waves whisper, "You've come a long way, baby," and I had to laugh. That's exactly what he would have said.

I marveled at how lighthearted I felt. The undertow of pain that had threatened to drown me at sea that day 43 years ago was so distant a memory today that it hardly seemed to be mine. Time is indeed a great healer, though when trauma narrows our window of tolerance we forget that.

I thought to myself, "Surely he'll have the last word." As I neared the end of my walk, I saw a well-bundled father and his young daughter sitting on a tarp, building an intricate sandcastle.

At that moment, I missed Dad terribly. I missed those memories we made when it was just the two of us. For decades, he hadn't been there to share the moments of glory or the moments of sorrow I had gone through since his death. I was struck more by the pain of his absence than the trauma of his violent end. Maybe today was my way of making a new memory or my chance to erase the last one I had when I was here. "I stay warm with my memories of you," I told him. "I have your green wool blanket folded over one of the chairs in the bedroom."

The father and daughter gathered their things and pulled up their tarp, leaving behind their creation. By the time I arrived at their spot, the fragile castle had been erased by the rising tide. Even so, I imagined they had made a memory sturdy enough to last in the years to come, as mine with Dad still do.

As I walked the beach on this cold, damp day all these years later I recalled Dad's last words to me long ago, "I love you, baby."

"I know, Dad," I replied now. "You're with me still. I love you, too."

It was hard to believe that day that there were times—even years—when my very survival seemed impossible. I couldn't imagine any other mental state than despair and any dreams I once had all but evaporated. If anyone tried to tell me that I would be where I am today or would achieve all that I have, I would not believe them.

That day, I left a lot of heavy baggage behind on the beach. If you are carrying Big Trauma baggage around with you, find your place to unburden yourself. For you, it may be the scene of an accident. Or, instead, it may be a park, a river, a cabin in the woods, or a big comfy chair. It might be a beautiful place where you shared sunrises or sunsets.

Wherever it is, go there. Promise yourself that you will not leave until you have achieved closure regarding your Big Trauma. Tell yourself this is the time when you pledge that you will leave the daily distractions of loss and sorrow behind and embrace where you are now. Stay as long as you need to, then walk away and go to your safest place to fall. I believe that every day we live there is the opportunity to make new memories that warm the heart, lift our spirits, and dull the remnants of trauma.

CHAPTER 17

Embracing Our Lives

"Not now, but now."

—M.F.K. FISHER

IF YOU ARE READING MY WORDS RIGHT NOW YOU WILL KNOW THAT dreams do come true, but often not until they—and we—are ready. Whatever dreams you may have, don't give up on them.

If you need help, ask for it. If you want answers, look for them. If you are confused, seek understanding. Whatever resistance you face to overcoming obstacles, please know that the reward of confronting and transcending them is worth the journey.

Somewhere out there, there are safe places and trustworthy people to comfort and heal you when you need it. Somewhere inside you, there is unconditional love and a compassionate heart for your own struggles.

Recently, Norm asked me, "Now that you have prepared your life to share, do you like yourself?" I answered yes and didn't have to even think about it. The self-acceptance that I have gained I want for you. I just hope it doesn't take you as long to find it as it took me.

When you arrive at the place you want to be, with the people you seek, doing what you desire, don't waste time judging the journey or the destination. And if someone asks you if you like yourself, I hope the answer is yes. Is it? If not, I hope you can get there without delay.

I wonder if you, like many of us, have put off doing something you have always dreamed of doing. Have you longed to take a solo journey around the world, travel to the Red Rocks outside Sedona, buy that weekend cabin? With all due humility, I say to you that there is no time like the present. If not now, then when?

That's one of the great mysteries of my journey. I ask myself often why I waited to clear my own path until my mother died. I had certainly made great strides while she was alive, but it wasn't until the final days of her life that I finally began to reclaim my own.

One of the happiest times I can remember was a sunny Saturday afternoon a few weeks before she died. Both of my children and several of my grandchildren crowded into the bedroom where Mom stayed now, too weak to get up or get dressed.

She was so proud that she had lived to see the birth of my fourth grandchild, who sat propped up by my mother's side, held lovingly close by my son. A special thing happened then that was noticed by me if not by others. When my infant granddaughter focused on Mom's face and put her little hand on her cheek, my mother smiled one of the most genuine smiles I had ever seen. She directed her gaze straight at me. There was so much love and laughter in that room that it crowded out any sadness that lay on the edges of the day.

In the last week of Mom's life, there is another day that stands out, when it was just the two of us and Mom was on hospice care and hadn't been out of bed for several weeks. I sat by the side of her bed and held her hand for hours. Sometimes she gripped my hand tightly, and at others, her hand went limp in mine. I had to make sure she hadn't slipped away altogether. Sometimes there were long silences as she drifted away from me. I would bring a straw close to her parched lips so she could take a sip of water. I'd run cool water on a washcloth and press it gently on her forehead.

She'd whisper, "I love you." At other times, she would say, "I'm sorry" or "I'm ready to go." All the years of pain between us melted away. In the end, we knew the love we were meant to have for each other from the beginning.

The last thing my mother whispered to me that day was, "You make me so happy." Then she took both my hands in hers. I remained by her side for an hour while I watched the sun glisten on the water and the boats gently bobbing as they sat moored to the docks that lined my mother's corner of the cove.

As dusk fell, I felt complete and at peace. I watched her drift off into a deep sleep. I whispered, "Goodbye," but she didn't seem to hear.

The bond between us was finally sealed by the shared expression of unconditional love. To paraphrase Dr. Hellinger: "To the extent that we reject our mothers, we reject ourselves. To the extent that we accept our mothers, we accept ourselves." I can't overstate the significance of this truism.

Now would be a good time for you to sit down with your journal, or just with yourself, to reflect on the nature of your own relationship with your mother. How would you describe the bond between you? Make a list of what you reject about your mother and why? Is there some way that you can come to accept her failings or shortcomings?

If your mother is still alive, is there something you can do to work through outstanding issues with her and come to a place of greater understanding and acceptance between you? If not, is there some personal work that you can do to heal the broken bond in your own psyche?

You might consider reading about the significance of the bond between mother and child in Dr. Hellinger's books or those of other experts in the field, or seek out practitioners of family constellation work to guide you.

On the Other Side

At this point in my life, I feel safely on the other side of the trauma. My family is slowly healing. The influence of inherited trauma is receding. We are beginning to take on new, more positive roles in each other's lives that are providing us with opportunities for healing. When we are together now, there is love without tension, laughter without reservation, and hopefulness about the future. I am optimistic that the dysfunction and the family inheritance have been mitigated and somehow resolved, at least for me.

There is no denying that the vast majority of my life is behind me. It's legitimate to ask myself what took me so long. Yet, I wonder, if I hadn't waited, who would I be now? If I had swiveled a little to the left or the right, my path would have been different and so would I. But can I say that different would have been better or worse, taken less time or more? I can't.

A life has so many moving parts that it's often difficult to keep them all balanced and moving at a steady pace. It's easy to look back and see our mistakes. It's harder to recognize and accept who we were and how we behaved at any given time or why we made the decisions we did. Can you give that forgiveness and acceptance to yourself? And if not now, then when?

As I began this journey, I would never have imagined for myself the unconditional love and peace of mind that are now mine. Life has exceeded all of my expectations. Each day has a mysterious and mystical element to it that I welcome. I see that the way my life has unfolded is different than I imagined. But I don't affix any judgment to how it's different than what I expected.

After all, I have long suspected that it is our expectations that fail us, not reality. All I do know is that I no longer live my life according to unrealistic expectations and I avoid taking actions or making decisions that I know I will regret.

When I survey my path through life, I now see what circumstances I actually could control. I wonder if I could have used my energy more judiciously, focusing on the areas I was truly able to impact and letting go of the rest. How much stress did I unnecessarily add to the journey?

I recognize now that the most control we have in life is over ourselves, our emotions and decisions, and even what we demand, both for and from ourselves. I look at the evolution of my work and I know for certain that it has mirrored my own evolution. I am grateful for the opportunity to grow and help others and for the resulting healing.

We are living in such uncertain times. Living in the moment and making the most of the time we have has never seemed so important.

I hope that you are able to look at those things that you have put off doing or saying or being. I hope you'll embrace the truths and changes that will enrich your life and bring you joy.

Barbara "Bobbi" Lambert, PhD

BARBARA "BOBBI" LAMBERT, PHD, IS A COFOUNDER OF CONFIDANTE, Inc., a San Francisco Bay Area human resources consulting company that specializes in creating workplace harmony and preventing and managing disruptive workplace behavior. She has a doctorate and a master's degree in Psychology. Since 1985, Dr. Lambert has worked with employers interested in the on-site management of individual performance and interpersonal problems, teamwork improvements, organizational development and change, stress, trauma, and violence. She has successfully facilitated, mediated, and resolved complex interpersonal and business conflicts to avoid critical incidents and costly litigation. Dr. Lambert has conducted research and developed best practice programs in the areas of hiring, performance management, retention, and workplace threats and violence. She spent seven years as the National Director of Training, Education, and Consultation at U.S. Behavioral Health, a national firm specializing in Employee Assistance, Substance Abuse, and Managed Mental Health Programs, and 15 years consulting to Wegmans Food Markets' Executive, Human Resources, and Asset Protection Divisions.

Dr. Lambert has extensive experience in the fields of workplace behavior, human resources management, hiring, training, organizational development, and strategic planning. She specializes in providing intervention services in complex and challenging personal and interpersonal relationships and situations that include executive coaching, mediation, anger management, group facilitation and interpersonal skill development, conflict management, workplace investigations and assessments, and critical incident prevention and management. Dr. Lambert, as the primary intervention expert, led a team of crisis management specialists in response to the July 1, 1993 shooting incident at the law firm of Pettit & Martin in San Francisco, where nine people were killed by a disgruntled client. As a respected lecturer and author, she has been a presenter at conferences on topics including Hiring and Retaining the Best, Workplace Violence—Lessons From the Trenches, Navigating the Tricky Waters of Workplace Investigations, Prevention and Resolution of "Hostile Workplace" Situations, Preventing Sexual Harassment in the Workplace, Turning Organizational Crisis to Productive Outcomes, Mental Health at Work, Workplace Stress and Trauma, and Chemical Dependency in the Workplace. Her articles and interviews have been published in *Business Week*, *The Associated Press*, *California Association of Workplace Investigators Journal*, *EAP Magazine*, *Workforce Magazine*, *HR Magazine*, *Bureau of National Affairs*, and *The Workplace Violence and Behavior Newsletter*.

Further Reading And References

Ariely, Dan (2008) *Predictably Irrational: The Hidden Forces that Shape Our Decisions*, Harper, An Imprint of HarperCollins Publishing

Ariely, Dan (2012) *The (Honest) Truth About Dishonesty: How We Lie to Everyone—Especially Ourselves*, Harper, An Imprint of HarperCollins Publishing

Assagioli, Roberto (1961) *Psychosynthesis: A Collection of Basic Writings*, An Esalen Book by Viking Press

Assagioli, Roberto (1973) *The Act of Will*, An Esalen Book by Viking Press

Cousineau, Phil (2011) *Beyond Forgiveness: Reflections on Atonement*, Jossey-Bass

Ferrucci, Piero (1982) *What We May Be: Techniques for Psychological and Spiritual Growth*, J.P. Tarcher Inc.

Ferrucci, Piero (2013) *Your Inner Will: Finding Personal Strength in Critical Times*, J.P. Tarcher Inc./Penguin Books

Fisher, M.F.K. (1947) *Not Now but Now*, New York Viking Press

Gardner, James C. (1999) *Overcoming Anxiety, Panic and Depression: New Ways to Regain Confidence*

Hellinger, Bert (2011) *Laws of Healing: Getting Well, Staying Well*, Hellinger Publications

Hellinger, Bert and Beaumont, Hunter (1991) *Touching Love: A Teaching Seminar*, Carl-Auer-Systeme Verlag

Jung, Carl Gustav (1956) *Modern Man in Search of a Soul*, Harcourt, Brace

Kubler-Ross, Elizabeth and Kessler, David (reprint 2007) *Five Stages of Grief*, Scribner Books Company

Manne, Joy and Hellinger, Bert (2009) *Family Constellations: A Practical Guide to Uncovering the Origins of Family Conflict*, North Atlantic Books

Merton, Thomas (1948) *The Seven Story Mountain: An Autobiography of Faith*, Harvest Books, Harcourt Press

Merton, Thomas (1958) *Thoughts in Solitude*, Farrar, Strauss, Giroux, New York

Merton, Thomas (2003) *The Inner Experience: Notes on Contemplation*, Harper One

Porges, Stephen W. (2017) *The Pocket Guide to the Polyvagal Theory: The Transformative Power of Feeling Safe*, W.W. Norton & Company

Rawlings, Emma Farr (2018) *The Divine Child: Your Soul's Inner Voice*, Waterside Press

Ruppert, Franz (2014) *Trauma, Fear and Love: How the Constellation of the Intention Supports Healthy Autonomy*, Green Balloon Publishing

Ruppert, Franz (2015) *Trauma, Bonding & Family Constellations: Understanding and Healing Injuries to the Soul*, Green Balloon Publishing

Ruppert, Franz (2018) *Who am I in a Traumatised and Traumatising Society?*, Green Balloon Publishing

Siegel, Daniel J. (2017) *Mind: A Journey to the Heart of Being Human*, W.W. Norton & Company

Wolynn, Mark (2016) *It Didn't Start With You: How Inherited Family Trauma Shapes Who We Are and How to End the Cycle*, Viking/Penguin Random House LLC

Other References and Resources

Confidante Intercommunications Systems, Inc.
www.confidante.com

The Alan Parsons Project (1984) Lyrics from "Days are Numbers" from the album *Vulture Culture*

National Council for Behavioral Health (2015) "Strengthening Personal and Community Resilience to Mitigate the Impact of Disaster Trauma"

Nalanda Institute, New York (2018) "Love's Brain: A Conversation with Stephen Porges with Joe Loizzo"

American Psychological Association (2020) "Pandemics: Covid-19 Information and Resources, Special Section"

Harvard Business Review (March 2020) "That Discomfort You're Feeling Is Grief, an Interview with David Kessler" by Scott Berinato

The Institute of Psychosynthesis, founded by Dr. Roberto Assagioli (opened in Rome in 1926 and reopened in Florence in 1946)

Psychosynthesis Workbook (1978) "Who Am I" by B. Carter-Harr

The Anxiety Toolbox Program (2020) by Dr. James Gardner

Acknowledgments

I WANT TO FIRST AND FOREMOST ACKNOWLEDGE AND THANK NORM, whose unconditional love taught me to love myself and others, whose love of writing became mine, whose belief that I am a writer encouraged my own passion and confidence. He has also been patient with me and served as muse, reader, editor, and enthusiastic, unwavering supporter throughout the writing of this book and all of the unfinished, incomplete manuscripts that came before. He brought meaning and peace of mind at a time when I had none and has always had my back in all things. He's my safe place to fall.

I want to thank and acknowledge my dear friend and life coach, Gita, who gave me a safe place to fall in Sedona and had the wisdom to introduce me to Family Constellation Theory and practice, which allowed me to heal inherited trauma that I didn't even know was at play. Gita also read, edited, and advised me on near-weekly marathon phone conversations as I worked my way from the original concept and draft to the final version of this book.

Thanks to Phil who edited and advised and provided me with such positive and profound feedback. He inspired me to take a deeper dive into myself and the ways in which my writing reflected unfinished psychological work with my family and helped me exit the perpetrator-victim cycle where I was stuck. His writing philosophy and his book on forgiveness and atonement helped me come to a more peaceful place with myself and my history. He inspired me to find my way to publishing and never give up on my dream.

I want to thank my coach and publisher, Catherine, and her professional editing and publishing team at Modern Wisdom Press. They helped me turn what started as a memoir into what is called "transformational nonfiction" so that I could turn my life and experience into an inspirational guidebook for others. It was a challenging process but well worth it if it serves others who have experienced trauma and are still looking for safe places to land and heal.

I also want to thank my dear friend Emma, who inspired me through her own writing and publication. She also had the wisdom to introduce me to Catherine. We have known each other since our graduate school days, and to this day, she continues to guide me and create a safe place for truth and healing.

My gratitude extends as well to my counselor, Peter, who helped me through the dark places where my trauma psyche lay hidden and that my writing uncovered. He provided acceptance, compassion, and understanding in a safe, therapeutic setting. I would read my writing to him chapter by chapter and he would, in turn, read my emotions and guide me through the wounded parts of me and into the bright sunshine of today. Thank you for that and for introducing me to Porges' Polyvagal Theory and Franz Ruppert's writing.

Thank You

I thank you, my readers, for sharing my journey with me throughout the pages of this book. I am so grateful that you have read my book. I have revealed a great deal about my story, trauma, understanding, and healing. I've encouraged you to reflect on the traumas of your life and those close to you. I hope that in some small way I have provided you with some solace and a safe place to explore the possibilities that exist beyond the traumas that all too often define our lives.

I invite you to reach out to me if you are interested in learning more about my work and how we might work together in the future. You can read more about my professional life at www.confidante.com and email me at info@confidante.com. I will do my best to respond. You can also connect with me on LinkedIn. I invite you to kindly review my book on Amazon as well.